Fatty liver diet

Charles Thompson

Copyright© 2021by Charles Thompson

The presentation of the information is without contract or any type of guarantee assurance. The trademarks that are used are without any consent, and the publication of the trademark is without permission or backing by the trademark owner. All trademarks and brands within this book are for clarifying purposes only and are the owned by the owners themselves, not affiliated with this document.

Index

Fatty liver diet

Introduction

The liver, with its 1500 grams, is the largest gland in our body. Its functions are multiple and largely essential. Among these, a role of primary importance is played by the sorting and synthesis of fats. In particular conditions of functional overload, this metabolism can go into crisis, favoring the accumulation of triglycerides inside the hepatocytes. When the liver's lipid content exceeds 5% of its weight, it is referred to as fatty liver or, more commonly, fatty liver.

About 20-40% of American adults "suffer" from fatty liver disease. In itself, this disorder is not an actual disease but a simple metabolic disadvantage, often asymptomatic. Only when the liver is very involved with steatosis, the patient can feel a sense of discomfort, a slight tenderness localized in the right quadrant of the abdomen. The liver shows signs of the disorder only in very advanced stages. What the patient refers typically to as a pain in the liver turns out to be, in many cases, simple pain in the intestine or the gallbladder (gallbladder). Precisely by its asymptomaticity, more than 90% of people with fatty liver occasionally discover this disorder. This is why hepatic steatosis is often discovered by chance, during an ultrasound performed for simple control or another pathology.

However, slight increases in transaminases (enzymes present in the blood) are often the fatty liver indicator. Simultaneously, fatigue, weakness, sudden weight loss can be signs of more advanced disease. The therapeutic approach for fatty liver consists of lifestyle modification and proper nutrition. In this guide, we will illustrate the recommended and non-recommended foods, as well as numerous recipes.

We remind you that it is essential to contact your family doctor, who will be able to advise you on the right treatment and diet.

Chapter 1:What is fatty liver?

For hepatic steatosis, we mean the infiltration of fat into the liver, mainly in the form of triglycerides, accumulated in the liver cells in such quantities as to exceed 5% of the liver's weight. There are two types of fatty liver disease: non-alcoholic and alcoholic.

Non-alcoholic fatty liver disease is a condition that includes a broad spectrum of liver diseases: from already advanced clinical pictures such as non-alcoholic steatohepatitis, characterized by necroinflammation and fibrosis of various degrees, to the risk of developing liver cirrhosis and related complications for health. It is characterized by a clinical picture similar to alcoholic steatosis, but it develops in people whose alcohol consumption is absent or negligible. It is probably the most common and frequent form of liver disease: it is estimated that about 20% of the adult population is affected by non-alcoholic fatty liver disease, but it is estimated that its prevalence in the obese population increases to 60-95% and the probability of passing from fatty tissue to steatohepatitis (a pathology at risk of developing into liver cirrhosis) increases with increase in the degree of obesity. The pediatric population data show how this pathology affects up to 17% of healthy children and 50% of obese children, thus representing an emerging problem even in developmental age. In turn, non-alcoholic fatty liver disease is divided into:

a) primary, associated with the metabolic syndrome (defined as the combination of different cardiovascular risk factors depending on the criterion considered, including obesity, dyslipidemia, increased waist circumference, hypertension, hypertriglyceridemia, hyperglycemia, and low HDL cholesterol values). At least one diagnostic criterion of metabolic syndrome is present in 90% of non-alcoholic fatty liver disease subjects. The prevalence of the syndrome in question increases with increasing body mass index (BMI). Furthermore, from a clinical perspective, the steatotic liver is an indicator of increased risk for diabetes mellitus and cardiovascular events.

b) secondary, which develops in people undergoing surgery and following severe low-calorie diets, protracted parenteral nutrition, etc.

Alcoholic steatosis, on the other hand, occurs in most heavy drinkers but is reversible when alcohol consumption is discontinued and is not believed to be a condition inevitably preceding the development of alcoholic hepatitis or cirrhosis. Dietary treatments are primarily aimed at removing risk factors. Being steatosis and steatohepatitis associated with alterations in glucose and lipid metabolism, obesity, and insulin resistance, a diet that considers the recommendations inherent in the guidelines for a healthy diet and a lifestyle change aimed at reduction of sedentary lifestyle represents the first and most important therapy. Nutritional goals must reduce insulin resistance and triglyceride values, improve metabolic parameters, and protect the liver from oxidative stress.

In the case of metabolic alterations and obesity, more detailed programs can be associated to gradually achieve adequate weight loss to be maintained over time. Weight loss of 10% of the starting weight can be associated with a normalization of liver enzymes and a decrease in hepatomegaly. Even a more modest weight loss (about 6%) can improve insulin resistance and liver fat content.

Abdominal fat: subcutaneous or visceral?

The people most at risk are certainly those who have visceral excess abdominal fat. Abdominal fat can be of two types, subcutaneous or visceral. The first, perhaps unaesthetic but not dangerous to health, is fat that has gone to localize at the peripheral level, in the layer that is directly under the skin. It visually creates the typical "rolls" that can be achieved. However, in the second case, fat occupies an internal and deep position in the abdominal cavity, localizing itself around the pancreas and liver. This type of fat is recognizable because it determines the presence of a swollen and tough belly, which you cannot reach with your hands. Over time, visceral fat comes from the organs, particularly the liver, causing hepatic steatosis. A specific concentration of fat within the liver is physiological. Still, when this exceeds 10-15%, it becomes pathological; we speak of "fatty liver," a condition that significantly increases the risk of cardiovascular and metabolic diseases.

When can we consider it a serious condition?

There are several stages of steatosis. The initial phase, absolutely asymptomatic, does not involve particular health risks, but, if neglected, it can evolve into advanced stages, which are those related to cardiovascular and metabolic risks. The phase following steatosis is non-alcoholic steatohepatitis, characterized, in addition to the accumulation of fat, by inflammatory processes that can lead to scarring and necrosis of the tissues and, in the most serious cases, to permanent damage with liver failure (cirrhosis) and, therefore, compromise in part or all of the functionality of the organ. In this stage, obvious symptoms may occur, such as discomfort and/or pain in the right side of the abdomen, fatigue, weakness, weight loss, itching, and swelling of the legs, ankles, and liver cirrhosis.

Chapter 2: Causes and symptoms

Causes

Fatty liver is caused by an excessive intake of alcohol, carbohydrates, dietary lipids, or an impaired ability to dispose of fat. The causes of hepatic steatosis are many and can give rise to the disease in an autonomous or multifactorial way; the most frequent are:

- obesity,
- type 2 diabetes,
- insulin resistance,
- hyperglycemia,
- hypertriglyceridaemia (elevated triglycerides in the blood),
- hypercholesterolemia (high cholesterol in the blood),
- high pressure.

Other risk factors also include:

- polycystic ovary syndrome (which in turn is linked to a high risk of diabetes and metabolic syndrome),
- sleep apnea syndrome,
- hypothyroidism,
- smoke.

The disorder is undoubtedly more common in adulthood (after the age of 50), but it can also affect children, especially if obese; according to some sources, it would be more common in men. A possible genetic predisposition is also recognized.

Symptoms

Usually, the affected patient does not manifest any symptoms in the early stages of steatosis, and the diagnosis is often made by chance during checks carried out for other reasons.

In people who also develop inflammation of the liver (steatohepatitis) and fibrosis, the following may occur:

- dull abdominal pain, in the right side,
- severe fatigue,
- unexplained weight loss,
- weakness.

In the case of cirrhosis, the symptoms become more evident and severe:

- yellowing of the skin and whites of the eyes,
- itch,
- swelling of the legs, ankles, feet or belly.

Complications

Non-alcoholic fatty liver diseases can undergo development in 4 phases, in which each step represents a more or less significant worsening of the pathology. Most people develop only the first stage, often without even knowing it, but the few who progress unfortunately experience potential permanent liver damage.
Steatosis (fatty liver): A largely harmless accumulation of fat in liver cells can be randomly diagnosed during ultrasound scans, often required for other reasons. It may affect up to one in three people.

Non-alcoholic steatohepatitis: a more severe form of steatosis that manifests itself in the presence of inflammation; it is estimated that it affects about 5% of the population.

Fibrosis occurs when persistent inflammation causes scar tissue to appear on the liver and near nearby blood vessels; however, the body can still function normally.

Cirrhosis: the most severe stage, which occurs after years of inflammation, and in which the liver shrinks and appears filled with scar tissue; this is permanent damage that can lead to liver failure (the liver stops functioning correctly) and liver cancer.

It can take years for fibrosis and cirrhosis to develop, but immediate lifestyle changes are imperative to prevent it from worsening.

The importance of early diagnosis

Early diagnosis is therefore of fundamental importance to avoid the disease's progression and prevent fearful complications. Since there are no symptoms initially, it can be handy to have an abdominal ultrasound scan, especially in cases where a healthy diet is not followed or in any case in the presence of metabolic diseases, such as diabetes. Blood tests can also help understand whether a fatty liver condition is developing, with even slight increases in transaminases, associated or not with high triglyceride values, especially if they are present simultaneously as fatigue, weakness, and weight loss.

Chapter 3: Lifestyle and Diet

The most important thing is to improve your lifestyle, absolutely losing weight if you are obese or overweight, practicing physical activity, and following a healthy and balanced diet. All of these factors can stop the disease's progression and improve the patient's state of health.

- In the case of overweight or obesity, it is necessary to eliminate the extra pounds and normalize the abdominal circumference, an indicator of the amount of fat deposited at the visceral level, mainly related to cardiovascular risk. Waist circumference values greater than 94 cm in men and 80 cm in women are associated with a "moderate risk," values greater than 102 cm in men, and 88 cm in women are associated with a "high risk."

- Avoid DIY diets! Too fast weight loss can lead to complications (accelerate the disease's progression and lead to the formation of gallstones). Furthermore, a too restricted diet prevents successful weight loss and increases the risk of regaining the lost pounds (yo-yo effect).

- In the case of metabolic alterations and obesity, more particular dietary programs can be associated, provided by the nutritionist, allowing them to gradually achieve an adequate weight loss to be maintained over time.

- Make your lifestyle more active. Give up the sedentary lifestyle! Go to work on foot, by bicycle or park far away, if you can avoid using the lift and take the stairs on foot, etc.

- Practice physical activity at least three times a week (ideally 300 minutes). The choice must always be made in the context of sports with aerobic characteristics (moderate intensity and long duration), such as cycling, aerobic gymnastics, walking at 4 km per hour, swimming, etc. These activities are more effective for eliminating excess fat.

- Do not smoke: Smoking is a cardiovascular risk factor.

- Check with your doctor for any other coexisting pathologies (e.g., arterial hypertension, diabetes mellitus, etc.).

- Read the products' food labels, especially to be sure of their content in sugars, saturated fats, and hydrogenated fats. Pay attention to the use of "sugar-free" products, as they are often rich in fat and consequently high in calories.

- Even if you are of average weight, it is good to monitor your body weight to prevent weight gains that favor fatty liver onset.

The role of nutrition

The first food advice in the fatty liver diet is to consume light meals, several times a day, containing all the nutrients in the right quantities and proportions ". These rules, which apply to all people, are fundamental in the patient with hepatic steatosis, to support the entire digestive process and avoid overloading the liver. Hence, "the three main meals, therefore breakfast, lunch, and dinner, which must be light and balanced, must always be accompanied by a mid-morning snack and two afternoon snacks.

General dietary recommendations

- Choose foods that are high in fiber and low in simple sugars;
- Choose foods with a low content of saturated fats and favor those with a higher content of monounsaturated and polyunsaturated fats;
- Cooking without added fats. Prefer simple cooking methods such as steam cooking, microwave, grill or plate, pressure cooker, etc. instead of frying, cooking in a pan or boiled meat;
- Avoid periods of prolonged fasting, eat regular meals. Prefer three main meals (breakfast, lunch, dinner) and two snacks a day to better control the sense of hunger / satiety and reduce glycemic peaks;

- On the advice of your doctor, it is possible to take supplements based on antioxidants, Omega-3 and vitamins, in particular vitamin E, vitamin C and vitamin D, but always in a controlled way to avoid the risk of hypervitaminosis;

FOOD NOT ALLOWED

- Spirits: liqueurs, alcoholic cocktails, etc.
- Alcohol, including wine and beer.
- Sweetened drinks such as cola, orange soda, tonic water, iced teas, but also fruit juices, as they naturally contain simple sugars (fructose) even if they bear the wording "no added sugar" on the package.
- White sugar and brown sugar to sweeten drinks, eventually replacing it with a zero-calorie sweetener.
- Jam and honey.
- Fruit in syrup, candied fruit, fruit mustard.
- Sweets and sweets such as cakes, pastries, biscuits, shortbreads, jellies, puddings, candies, etc.
- Baked products (eg crackers, breadsticks, taralli, croutons, biscuits, brioches, etc.) which, among the ingredients, carry the wording "vegetable fats" (unless otherwise specified, generally contain saturated vegetable oils such as palm and coconut).
- Fast-food foods rich in fat, also present in many industrially or artisanal prepared foods and in ready meals.
- Animal fats such as butter, lard, and cream.

- Animal offal
- Sausages with a high content of saturated fats,
  such as sausage in addition to the fatty parts of
  the meat (with visible fat).
- Mayonnaise, ketchup, mustard, barbecue sauce
  and other elaborate sauces.

FOODS ALLOWED WITH MODERATION

- Grapes, bananas, figs, persimmons and
  mandarins, as they are the most sugary fruits.
  Even dried and dried fruit should be consumed to
  a limited extent and in smaller portions than
  other types of fruit.
- Salt . It is a good idea to reduce the amount
  added to dishes during and after cooking and
  limit the consumption of foods that naturally
  contain high quantities (canned foods, nuts and
  meat extracts, sauces such as soy).
- Potatoes, which are not vegetables but important
  sources of starch. They are therefore to be
  consumed in place of bread, pasta, rice and
  cereals in general. They can be consumed
  occasionally as a substitute for the first course,
  but not fried.
- Sliced, once or twice a week as long as they are
  degreased. Among these, cooked ham, raw ham,
  speck, bresaola and sliced turkey or chicken are
  to be preferred.

- Cheeses, once or twice a week to replace the second dish. Among the fresh ones it is good to prefer those with low fat content, while among the aged cheeses those produced with milk that is partially decimated during processing.
- Polyunsaturated or monounsaturated vegetable oils such as extra virgin olive oil, rice oil or single seed oils: soy, sunflower, corn, peanut, etc. Due to their high calorie content, it is a good idea to use a teaspoon to control the quantities, avoiding pouring them directly from the bottle.
- Coffee . Some studies in the scientific literature show a protective effect on the liver, i.e. the ability to reduce the risk of non-alcoholic fatty liver disease. However, one must not overdo it. Two or three cups a day are fine, more could lead to various problems, including difficulty falling asleep, gastric upset and tachycardia.

ALLOWED AND RECOMMENDED FOODS

- Fish of all kinds, at least three times a week. Give preference to the blue one (e.g. herring, sardines, mackerel, anchovies, etc.) and salmon for their high content of omega 3 fatty acids.
- Raw and cooked vegetables to be consumed in large portions. The variety in the choice allows you to correctly introduce all the mineral salts, vitamins and antioxidants necessary for the health of the body. Some vegetables have a distinctly hepatic tropism, that is, they have a tonic and detoxifying action on the liver: artichokes and especially bitter herbs, such as chicory from Catalonia.
- Fruit, due to the high content of mineral salts, vitamins and antioxidants. It is best not to exceed two servings per day, as it naturally contains sugar (fructose). Prefer seasonal fruit and limit the sugary fruits previously mentioned to occasional consumption.
- Bread, pasta, rice, oats, barley, spelled and other complex carbohydrates, favoring wholemeal ones with a lower glycemic index.
- Skimmed or partially skimmed milk and yogurt.

- Meat, both red and white, coming from lean cuts and deprived of visible fat. Poultry should be eaten without the skin, because it is the part that provides the most fat.
- Legumes (beans, chickpeas, peas, broad beans, lentils, etc.), two to four times a week, fresh or dried, to be consumed as a main course.
- Water (at least 2 L per day), tea, herbal teas or infusions without adding sugar.
- Aromatic herbs to flavor dishes.

Diet plan example

Here is a diet plan for a man with the following features:

Gender: Male

Age: 40 years

Stature: 178.0cm

Constitution: Normal

Weight: 88.0Kg

Assessment: Overweight

Physiological weight desirable: 70kg

DIET EXAMPLE DAY 1

Breakfast

- Soy milk, enriched in calcium 300ml 1 cup
- Oat flakes 40g 8 tbsp

Snack 1

- Apple, with peel 200g 1 apple
- Rice cakes without salt 16g 2 cakes

Lunch

Pasta with tomato sauce

- wholemeal pasta 80g
- Tomato puree 100g
- Grated Parmesan 10g 2 tsp

Snack 2

- Oranges 300g 1 orange
- Natural yogurt, skimmed 120g 1 jar
- Rice cakes without salt 8g 1 cake

Dinner

- Boiled Beans 40 g

Grilled Polo Breast and Stewed Artichokes

- Chicken Breast 150g
- Artichokes 200g
- Wheat bread 30g 1 slice
- Extra virgin olive oil 15g 3 tsp

DIET EXAMPLE DAY 2

Breakfast

- Soy milk, enriched in calcium 300ml 1 cup
- Corn flakes 40g 8 tbsp

Snack 1

- Pear, with peel 200g 1 pear
- Rice cakes without salt 16g 2 cakes

Lunch

Risotto with Zucchini

- Rice, whole grain 80g
- Zucchini 100g
- Parmesan 10g 2 tsp

- Red cabbage 200g
- Wholemeal bread 30g 1 slice
- Extra virgin olive oil 15g 3 tsp

Snack 2

- Kiwi 200g 2 kiwis
- Natural yogurt, skimmed 120g 1 jar
- Rice cakes without salt 8g 1 cake

Dinner

Cooked chickpeas

- Chickpeas, dried 40g

Fillet of Sea Bass and Steamed Carrots

- Sea bass, fillets 150g
- Carrots 200g
- Wheat bread 30g 1 slice
- Extra virgin olive oil 15g 3 tsp

DIET EXAMPLE DAY 3

Breakfast

- Soy milk 300ml 1 cup
- Oats 40g 8 tbsp

Snack 1

- 1 Orange
- Rice cakes without salt 16g 2 cakes

Lunch

Soup (with Potatoes) and Barley

- Whole barley 50g
- Frozen vegetables (with potatoes) 300g
- Parmesan 10g 2 tsp

- Wholemeal bread 30g 1 slice
- Extra virgin olive oil 15g 3 tsp

Snack 2

- Pomegranate, peeled 100g 1 pomegranate
- Natural yogurt, skimmed 120g 1 jar
- Rice cakes without salt 8g 1 cake

Dinner

Boiled Lentils

- Lentils, dried 40g

Egg omelette, egg whites and spinach

- Whole egg 50g 1 chicken egg
- Egg whites 350g
- Spinach 200g

- Wheat bread 30g 1 slice
- Extra virgin olive oil 15g 3 tsp

DIET EXAMPLE DAY 4

Breakfast

- Soy milk 300ml 1 cup
- Whole grains 40g 8 tbsp

Snack 1

- Grapes 100g
- Rice cakes without salt 16g 2 cakes

Lunch

Potato, Rocket and Parsley Salad

- Potatoes 450g
- Rocket 100g
- Parsley (fresh) QB

- Wholemeal bread 30g 1 slice
- Extra virgin olive oil 15g 3 tsp

Snack 2

- Winter melon 300g 3 slices
- Natural yogurt, skimmed 120g 1 jar
- Rice cakes without salt 8g 1 cake

Dinner

Boiled peas

- Peas, dried 40g

Lean Milk Flakes with Fennel

- Light Milk Flakes 150g 1 jar
- Fennel 200g
- Wheat bread 30g 1 slice
- Extra virgin olive oil 15g 3 tsp

DIET EXAMPLE DAY 5

Breakfast

- Soy milk 300ml 1 cup
- Oat flakes 40g 8 tbsp

Snack 1

- Apple, with peel 200g 1 apple
- Rice cakes without salt 16g 2 cakes

Lunch

Pasta with Eggplant

- Wholemeal pasta 80g
- Eggplant 100g
- Parmesan10g 2 tsp

- Thistles 200g
- Wholemeal bread 30g 1 slice
- Extra virgin olive oil 15g 3 tsp

Snack 2

- Oranges 300g 1 orange
- Natural yogurt, skimmed 120g 1 jar
- Rice cakes without salt 8g 1 cake

Dinner

Boiled Beans

- Dried beans 40g

Grilled Veal Steak and Stewed Artichokes

- Veal, "walnut" cut 150g
- Artichokes 200g

- Wheat bread 30g 1 slice
- Extra virgin olive oil 15g 3 tsp

DIET EXAMPLE DAY 6

Breakfast

- Soy milk 300ml 1 cup
- Corn flakes 40g 8 tbsp

Snack 1

- Pear, with peel 200g 1 pear
- Rice cakes without salt 16g 2 cakes

Lunch

Pumpkin Risotto

- Rice, whole grain 80g
- Pumpkin 100g
- Parmesan 10g 2 tsp

- Broccoli 200g
- Wholemeal bread 30g 1 slice
- Extra virgin olive oil 15g 3 tsp

Snack 2

- Kiwi 200g 2 kiwis
- Natural yogurt, skimmed 120g 1 jar
- Rice cakes without salt 8g 1 cake

Dinner

Chickpeas boiled

- Chickpeas, dried 40g

Fillet of Sea Bream and Steamed Beets

- Sea bream, fillets 150g
- Beets 200g

- Wheat bread 30g 1 slice
- Extra virgin olive oil 15g 3 tsp

DIET EXAMPLE DAY 7

Breakfast

 Soy milk, 300ml 1 cup

- Oats 40g 8 tbsp

Snack 1

- 1 Orange
- Rice cakes without salt 16g 2 cakes

Lunch

Potato puree with spelled

- Potatoes 300g
- Spelled 30g
- Parmesan 10g 2 tsp
- Wholemeal bread 30g 1 slice
- Extra virgin olive oil 15g 3 tsp

Snack 2

- Pomegranate, peeled 100g 1 pomegranate
- Natural yogurt, skimmed 120g 1 jar
- Rice cakes without salt 8g 1 cake

Dinner

Boiled Lentils

- Lentils, dried 40g

Egg omelette, egg whites and chicory

Whole egg 50g 1 chicken egg

- Egg whites 350g
- Chicory 200g
- Wheat bread 30g 1 slice
- Extra virgin olive oil 15g 3 tsp

Chapter 4: Breakfast

1) Crêpes of chickpea flour with cabbage and fermented cashew nuts

Ingredients:

For the crêpes:

- **280 g of chickpea flour**
- **500 ml of warm water**
- **40 g of extra virgin olive oil**
- **4 g cumin seeds**
- **4 g sage**
- **8 g of whole salt**
- **10 cabbage leaves.**

For the cashew spread:

- **150 g raw cashews**
- **20 g white miso**
- **8 g lemon juice**
- **10 g nutritional yeast**
- **3 g of whole salt**
- **3 g yellow mustard powder**
- **water q.s.**

For the crêpes: with the help of a whisk, mix the chickpea flour, water, and 20 g of extra virgin olive oil. Leave to rest for at least 8 hours. Then pick up the dough and season it with a mix obtained by blending the cumin, sage, and salt. Mix well. Heat a non-stick or iron pot well, pour a teaspoon of sunflower oil, and distribute it well over the entire surface. Pour a ladle of batter, cook it until it comes off, then turn it over and cook it on the other side as well.

When it is ready, place it on absorbent food paper and proceed with the dough. Cut the cabbage leaves thin. Heat a wok-like pan with the remaining extra virgin olive oil. Sauté the cabbage for a few minutes, add salt and let the vegetation water evaporate and it will come out. Keep them aside. For the spread: soak the cashews for 12 hours at room temperature, changing the water at least a couple of times. After that, rinse them well and put them in a blender along with all the ingredients. Blend until the mixture is creamy and without lumps. Serve the crêpes with the cabbage, a few flakes of cashew spread, and grated black pepper.

2) Chocolate, almond, nut and coconut cookies

Ingredients:
- **100 g of dark chocolate**
- **50 g of shelled almonds**
- **50 g of walnut kernels**
- **30 g of shredded coconut**
- **50 g of whole coconut sugar**
- **1 egg white whipped until stiff**
- **the peel of 1 organic orange**
- **1 pinch of salt**

Put the diced chocolate and the other dry ingredients, including the orange peel, in the mixer. Blend everything for a few minutes until it is reduced to a powder. You will get a rather lumpy mixture. Meanwhile, whip the egg white until stiff and add it to the dough, mixing carefully. Using a spoon, form balls of the mixture and place them on a baking tray lined with parchment paper. Try to distance them from each other because they will widen during cooking. Bake the cookies at 150 ° for 25 minutes. Let them cool before removing them.

3)   Stuffed chickpea flour pancakes

Ingredients:
- 3 heaping tablespoons of spelled flour
- 2 heaping tablespoons of corn starch
- 3 heaping tablespoons of chickpea flour
- 2 tablespoons of oil and 1 pinch of salt
- 1 pinch of nutmeg
- 300 ml of partially skimmed milk

For the stuffing
- 1 small thistle (about 200 g) already cleaned
- 1 slice of clean pumpkin
- ½ small leek
- 2 teaspoons of flour
- 2 teaspoons of lemon juice
- 4 tablespoons of oil and 1 pinch of salt

For the batter: dissolve the flour and starch in a little milk, then gradually pour the remaining liquid and oil, beating with a whisk. When the cream is thick and fluid, add the salt and nutmeg. Let it sit for 20-30 minutes.

For the filling: blanch the thistle in 500 ml of water where you have diluted the lemon and flour. Wash the leek and slice it thinly. Sauté it in a pan with 1 tablespoon of oil and 3 of water for 4-5 minutes, then add the coarsely grated pumpkin and the shredded thistle. After another 4-5 minutes turn off the heat. Mix the batter. Just grease a non-stick pan and pour a ladle of the mixture into a thin layer. Cook the crepes for a few minutes on both sides. Stuff them and close them in a bundle. Serve hot.

4) Buckwheat pancakes with nettle sauce

Ingredients:
- **250 g of buckwheat flour**
- **150 g of nettle tops**
- **400 ml of soy milk**
- **3 tablespoons of white flour**
- **oil**
- **salt**

Put the flour in a bowl with the water needed to have a semi-fluid batter. Add salt, stir and let it rest for 30 minutes. Wash the nettles and blanch them for 5 minutes in a little salted water. Remove them with a slotted spoon and set them aside. Measure out 100 ml of their liquid (save the rest for other preparations). First, toast the white flour in a saucepan; first, pour the hot nettle water and then, always stirring and, little by little, the previously heated milk. Let the sauce thicken over low heat, then add the coarsely chopped nettles. Season with salt and season with a tablespoon and a half of oil. Heat a little oil in a pan and cook a ladle of batter at a time until you have not too thin crepes. Serve with the nettle sauce.

5)   Savory pie with potatoes and creamy mushrooms

Ingredients:

- **250 g of wholemeal flour**

- **3 tablespoons of sourdough**

- **soya milk**

- **1 teaspoon of brown sugar**

- **2 tablespoons of oil**

- **6 medium potatoes**

- **200 g of mushrooms**

- **100 g of vegetable cream**

- **150 g of ricotta**

- **2 cloves of garlic**

- **1 teaspoon of marjoram**

- **2 teaspoons of sweet paprika**

- **sea salt**

Mix the flour with the sourdough, a little salt, and the lukewarm milk necessary to have a firm and homogeneous dough. Knead it for a long time on a table, wrap it into a ball and let it rise in a warm place for 4-5 hours.

Meanwhile, wash the potatoes and steam them with the peel. While these are getting warm, peel the mushrooms and stew them in a pan with minced garlic, paprika, marjoram, and a little salt. When soft, add the cream and crumbled goat cheese. Peel the potatoes and cut them into slices about 1 cm thick. Roll out two thirds of the dough and use it to line a floured, rectangular, or round, high mold. Spread the potatoes inside, cover with mushrooms. Roll out the rest of the dough so that it covers the entire surface. Seal the edges well, brush with a little warm milk and bake at 180 degrees for 30-35 minutes. Serve the cake hot.

6)   Energy cookies with oats and raisins

Ingredients:
- **300 g of rolled oats**
- **100 g of raisins**
- **the grated zest of a lemon**
- **the zest of a grated orange**
- **150 g of rice malt**
- **a teaspoon of ground cinnamon**
- **a teaspoon of vanilla powder**
- **apple juice to taste**

First, soak the raisins in warm water for about 15 minutes, turn on the oven at 180 ° and prepare a pan lined with parchment paper to lay the biscuits to cook them. Once this is done, you can dedicate yourself to the dough, starting with toasting the oat flakes in a hot pan for a few minutes, stirring often. Place them still hot in a large bowl in which you will add the grated citrus peel, cinnamon, vanilla powder, and finally, the well squeezed raisins. At this point, add the malt to the mixture; knead with your hands with the help of a little apple juice (just enough to be able to work the dough without making it too liquid). You can proceed by taking some of the dough to form balls that you will crush in your hands to give it the classic shape of a round biscuit. During this step, you can help yourself by wetting your hands with water. Place each biscuit in the pan and bake for about 10-15 minutes. Remove the pan from the oven and let the cookies cool. When they are cold, you can store them in an airtight jar, where they will keep well for a whole week.

7)   Omelette with potatoes and onions

Ingredients:
- **800 g of potatoes**
- **6 eggs**
- **2 onions**
- **2 cloves of garlic**
- **2 tablespoons of oil**
- **1 pinch of nutmeg**
- **1 pinch of parsley**
- **1 pinch of chives**
- **pepper**
- **salt**

Finely slice the onions and garlic. Wash and peel the potatoes and cut them into cubes. Fry the onions and garlic in a pan with olive oil and water, add the potatoes, and cook them until tender. Season with the chopped parsley and chives and mix well. Beat the eggs, add the grated nutmeg to taste, and pour the mixture over the potatoes. When the eggs have hardened, turn the omelette and finish cooking on the other side. Serve immediately.

8) Oat porridge with chocolate, cashew and orange

Ingredients:
- **about 10 tablespoons of oat flakes**
- **a few pinches of ground cinnamon**
- **a few pinches of vanilla powder**
- **2 tablespoons of rice syrup**
- **6-7 cashews**
- **dark chocolate to taste**
- **almond milk**
- **a slice of orange**

Put the oat flakes in a bowl, then pour enough milk to cover them abundantly. Let it rest in the fridge overnight. The next morning add the cinnamon, vanilla, rice syrup and mix well. Add more milk if necessary. Complete with crumbled or chopped cashews, dark chocolate into small pieces, and a slice of orange. Consume the porridge immediately.

9) Plum gluten-free muffins

Ingredients:
- **300 g of cooked prunes**
- **4 eggs**
- **150 g of brown sugar**
- **190 g of potato starch**
- **200 g of rice flour**
- **1 vanilla pod**

Whisk the whole eggs with the sugar and the seeds of the vanilla pod. Add the starch, flour, and plums with their liquid to the mixture. Mix well and arrange everything in

lightly oiled cups or silicone muffin molds; you should get
7-10 muffins depending on the molds' size. Bake in the
oven at 180-190 ° for about 25 minutes, or until it comes
out dry by inserting a toothpick inside the cake.

10) Pancakes without butter

Ingredients:
  - **Low-fat white yogurt 125 g**
  - **00 flour 150 g**
  - **Skimmed milk 200 g**
  - **Eggs 1**
  - **Powdered yeast for cakes 8 g**
  - **Extra virgin olive oil q.s.**

Start by placing the egg in a bowl and beating it with a
whisk. When it is light and fluffy, add the milk slowly and,
continue to beat, add the yogurt. Then add, passing it
through a sieve, the flour, and the baking powder.
Proceed by mixing carefully, with gentle movements from
the bottom to the top, to not disassemble the mixture,
until you get a smooth and homogeneous batter. Cover
with cling film, and place it in the fridge to rest for about
30 minutes. After this time, recover the batter and heat a
non-stick pan with a drizzle of oil over medium heat. Pour
a spoonful of batter into the center of the pan, letting it
spread by itself. After a few minutes, when small bubbles
begin to bloom on the surface, it is time to turn the
pancake with the help of a spatula. So cook it for another
minute and when it's ready, place it on a plate. Continue
like this until the batter is used up. Serve your butter-free
pancakes with honey!

11) Lentil crepes

Ingredients:
- **100-120 of cooked and well dried lentils**
- **3 tablespoons of flour**
- **100-120 ml of oat milk**
- **2 teaspoons of turmeric**
- **salt and black pepper**
- **oil**

For the filling:
- **tomato sauce**

Mix the cooled lentils with turmeric, a little salt, and black pepper. Dilute the flour in the vegetable milk. Add salt and gradually pour the mixture over the lentils. Mix well. Heat a small non-stick pan with a thin layer of oil and pour half of the dough at a time. Cook each crepe on both sides for a few minutes until it is golden brown. Serve the pancakes hot, sprinkled with a drizzle of oil.

12) Kamut flour biscuits

Ingredients:
- **250 g of kamut flour**
- **150 g of maple syrup**
- **50 g of chopped and toasted almonds**
- **70 ml of corn oil**
- **50 g of raisins**
- **50 g of unsweetened cocoa powder**
- **20 g of yeast**
- **200 ml of warm water**
- **1 teaspoon of vanilla**
- **the grated peel of ½ orange**
- **1 pinch of salt**

In a bowl, combine the oil and maple syrup, mixing well. Gather the dry ingredients in a bowl: the flour, the chopped almonds, the unsweetened cocoa, the baking powder, the salt, and the vanilla, mix them evenly and add the raisins, water, and the mixture with the syrup. 'Maple. Work with your hands until you get a soft and smooth dough: lifting a bit of the dough with one hand and letting it fall slowly. Pour some of the dough into the pastry bag and squeeze to form corrugated discs on the pan (space the cookies apart, so they have room to rise). Bake the cookies in the oven at 200 ° for 20 minutes. Let them cool and serve them.

Chapter 5: Snacks, appetizers and side dishes

1) Brussels sprouts with pears and walnuts

Ingredients
- 350 g of Brussels sprouts
- 40 g of leek
- 1 small pear
- 60 g of shelled walnuts
- 2 juniper berries
- salt
- 4 tablespoons of oil

Clean and wash the vegetables. Remove the most damaged leaves from the sprouts and divide them into four wedges; add them to the finely sliced leek, which you will dry for 5 minutes in a pan with 2 tablespoons of oil, half a glass of water, and the juniper. Cut the pear into cubes and coarsely chop the walnuts; add them to the mixture and continue cooking for another 3 minutes. Before removing from the heat, season with salt, season with the remaining oil, and stir.

2) Broccoli with miso sauce and nuts

Ingredients:
- **2-3 broccoli tops**
- **80 g of walnuts**
- **2 tablespoons of miso**
- **about 1 cm of ginger root**

Cut and wash the broccoli tops and place them in the steamer basket, adding a pinch of salt. Cook in a covered pot until the broccoli is tender but still bright green. Meanwhile, toast the walnuts in the oven at 180 ° until they are fragrant. Let them cool down. Chop them coarsely by hand to prevent them from releasing too much oil, and then grind them in a mixer with miso and water or vegetable broth, just enough to obtain a smooth cream. Flavor with the ginger juice, obtained by squeezing the grated root. Serve the vegetables with the sauce.

3)   Sweet and sour stewed pumpkin

Ingredients:
- **3 cups of chopped pumpkin**
- **2 tablespoons of extra virgin olive oil**
- **chopped sage to taste**
- **water q.s.**
- **2 tablespoons of rice vinegar**
- **salt**

Heat the oil in a pot with the chopped sage and rosemary, then add the pumpkin, a little salt and sauté for a few minutes. Add a little water and vinegar, cover, and let it simmer over low heat for about 15-20 minutes until the pumpkin is tender.

4)   Quick pizzas

Ingredients:
For the dough
- **200 g of finely ground millet**
- **200 g of rice flour**
- **3 tablespoons of oil**
- **1 teaspoon of salt**
- **1 tablespoon yeast**
- **1 tablespoon of sesame and flax seeds**

For the filling:
- **500 g of clean pumpkin**
- **1 sprig of sage**
- **1 sprig of rosemary**
- **2 tablespoons of oil**

For the mini pizzas: Finely chop the seeds. Combine them with the other ingredients in a large bowl and knead with your hands to get a soft and homogeneous mixture. Let it rest for about 1 hour. For the filling. Cut the pumpkin into cubes, sprinkle with chopped sage and rosemary. Cook it in steam or the oven for 15-20 minutes, let it cool, and season with oil. Blend it until you have a cream, helping you if needed with a little water. Roll out the not too thin dough with a rolling pin and cut out discs with the help of a glass; place them on a baking sheet lined with parchment paper and cover with the cream. Bake at 170 degrees for about 15 minutes.

5)   Mushrooms with orange spinach

Ingredients:
- **400 g of fresh spinach leaves**
- **150 g of champignon mushrooms**
- **2 large handfuls of shelled almonds**
- **the juice of 1 blond orange**
- **oil**
- **white pepper, to taste**
- **pink Himalayan salt, to taste**

Clean the spinach and the mushrooms, which you will then have to slice thinly. Put the vegetables in a bowl with the peeled and chopped almonds and mix well. Season with orange juice, oil, a few pinches of Himalayan salt, and freshly ground pepper. Stir again and serve.

6) Quinoa with roasted carrots

Ingredients:

• 250 g of quinoa

• 4-5 carrots

• 4 shallots

• 1/2 tablespoon of cumin

• 1/2 tablespoon of turmeric

• 1 handful of toasted pine nuts

• 1 handful of parsley and very finely chopped celery

• extra virgin olive oil

• salt and pepper

Peel the shallots and halve them; cut the carrots in four lengthwise and then into chunks. Put the vegetables in a pan seasoned with oil, cumin, and salt. Bake at 180 degrees for about 30 minutes, turning them now and then until they are well roasted. Meanwhile, wash the quinoa well in cold water, drain it in a tightly meshed colander and rinse again; drain well and dry briefly in a pan with two tablespoons of oil, turmeric, and pepper. Pour in boiling water equal to double the quinoa's volume, add salt, cover, and cook over very low heat for 15-20 minutes until the liquid is completely absorbed.

Shell the quinoa well and mix it with the vegetables, also collecting their cooking juices, with the pine nuts, celery, and parsley. Serve immediately.

7)   Carrot puree with green olives

Ingredients:
- **500 g of carrots**
- **1 teaspoon of paprika**
- **2 teaspoons of cumin**
- **3 tablespoons of rice vinegar**
- **2 minced garlic cloves**
- **1 tablespoon of oil**
- **grated ginger juice**
- **green olives for garnish**
- **salt and pepper**

Peel and cut the carrots into rings and place them in a steamer basket. Cook them, covered, in a saucepan with lightly salted boiling water. After about ten minutes, check that they are soft. Blend them with the rest of the ingredients and a little cooking water to obtain a puree's consistency. Let the puree rest for a couple of hours so that the flavors blend. If you prefer, put it in the fridge for a while. Serve at room temperature or slightly chilled.

8)   Eggplant and tofu meatballs

Ingredients:
- **100 g of tofu**
- **1 large eggplant**
- **1 clove of garlic**
- **2 sprigs of parsley**
- **1 tablespoon of flour**
- **4 tablespoons of breadcrumbs**
- **salt**
- **oil to taste**

Cook the whole eggplant in the oven; once cooked, sauté its pulp in a pan in a garlic sauce. Season with salt and add the crumbled tofu. Mix the ingredients, if necessary, with a little flour. Complete the preparation with chopped parsley. Prepare meatballs the size of an apricot, dip them in breadcrumbs, bake them or fry them in a pan, according to preference.

9) Spinach in a pan with dried fruit

Ingredients:

- **500 g of spinach**

- **50 g of dried apples**

- **50 g of raisins**

- **a little pine nuts**

- **1 clove of garlic**

- **extra virgin olive oil as needed**

- **Salt to taste**

Soak the apples and raisins for about 20 minutes in warm water. Clean and wash the spinach. Blanch them in lightly salted water for a few minutes. Drain them by squeezing them well, and cut them coarsely. Fry the garlic in a pan greased with oil, add the spinach, and after a while, the raisins and well-squeezed apples, pine nuts, and salt. Let it cook over high heat for a few minutes, season with salt, and serve the spinach hot.

10) Rice and zucchini croquettes with saffron sauce

Ingredients:

For the croquettes:

- 350 g of rice

- 850 ml of water

- 800 g of zucchini

- 2 tablespoons of oil

- 1 teaspoon of salt

- 1 bunch of parsley

- 1 clove of garlic

- salt and pepper

For the saffron sauce:

- 250 ml of soy milk

- 30 ml of oil

- 30 g of rice flour

- 1 sachet of saffron

Brown the chopped garlic and parsley in a little oil. Add and stew the sliced zucchini with salt and pepper for 10 minutes. Puree about 1/3 of the zucchini. Wash the rice, drain it and cook it in salted water, covered and without stirring, for about 35 minutes.

Season the rice with the salt, the zucchini not pureed, stir, and continue cooking for another 5 minutes. Let it cool, then form some meatballs that you will bake in the oven at 200 ° for about 15-20 minutes. To prepare the sauce, brown the flour in a saucepan with the oil, then add the milk. Bring to a boil and let it thicken over low heat, stirring with a whisk. Salt and add the saffron and the zucchini puree.

11) Rice balls with broccoli and almond pesto

Ingredients:
For the stuffing
• **leftover already seasoned rice, or other cereal.**
If you use leftover rice, millet, amaranth and
quinoa, the recipe is also suitable for celiacs.
• **extra virgin olive oil or seeds for frying**

For the batter
• **chickpea flour**
• **water q.s.**
• **a pinch of salt**
• **breadcrumbs**

For the broccoli and almond pesto
• **half a fresh broccoli**
• **80 g of almonds**
• **the juice of half a lemon**
• **a clove of garlic**
• **a large tuft of fresh parsley**
• **Salt to taste.**
• **extra virgin olive oil as needed**

Cut your broccoli into small pieces and steam it or cook it in a pot in hot water for a maximum of 10 minutes. Put it in the blender and add the remaining ingredients: the garlic clove into small pieces, the parsley, the lemon juice, the almonds, the salt, and the olive oil. Blend vigorously, help yourself using a little water if necessary (the one used for cooking broccoli, for example), taste, and season with salt. Put the pesto in a large bowl and let the ingredients rest.

At this point, we proceed with the preparation and cooking of the meatballs. In a bowl, mix the chickpea flour with water, avoiding the formation of lumps. Mix vigorously until you get a thick and homogeneous batter. Add a pinch of salt. Prepare a dish with the center's breadcrumbs: you can make your breading even tastier by adding chopped aromatic herbs, garlic or onion, sesame seeds, or chopped hazelnuts. With wet hands, take some leftover rice and form a ball to dip into the batter first and then pass it into the breadcrumbs. Repeat the operation until the dough is used up.

Prepare a pot with a high bottom and put the oil to heat. Once the temperature is reached, start frying your meatballs for a few minutes until they are golden, and place them in a dish lined with absorbent paper. Take a serving dish, place your hot and crunchy meatballs in the center, bring to the table and serve them accompanied by the broccoli and almond pesto sauce. Delicious!

12) Fennel in orange cream

Ingredients:
- **2 medium fennel**
- **1 cup of cashews**
- **125 ml of orange juice**
- **2 teaspoons of dried mint**
- **1 pinch of chilli**
- **1 tablespoon of oil**
- **½ teaspoon of salt**
- **1 teaspoon of agave syrup**

Wash the fennel, cut them into four parts, and, using a mandolin, slice them finely. Sprinkle it with salt and let it rest. Meanwhile, prepare the cream. Put the cashews in the blender with the orange juice, mint, chili pepper, oil, salt, and agave syrup and mix until the mixture is fluid and without lumps. Drain the fennel water and season with the cream.

Chapter 6: Soups and salads

1) Oat milk mushroom cream

Ingredients:
- **2 shallots**
- **2 tablespoons of flour**
- **400 ml of vegetable broth**
- **200 ml of oat milk**
- **400 g of mushrooms**
- **20 g of dried porcini mushrooms**
- **½ teaspoon of marjoram**
- **1 tablespoon of chopped parsley**
- **2 tablespoons of oil**
- **100 g of oat flakes**
- **salt**

Rinse the dried mushrooms and soak them in hot water for 30 minutes. Filter the liquid and squeeze the porcini mushrooms, then cut them up. Spread the flakes in a single layer on a baking sheet lined with baking paper, bake them at 180 ° and toast them for 10 minutes, turning them now and then. Let them cool. Meanwhile, you have cleaned the mushrooms with a damp cloth and sliced them. Chop the shallots and put them in a pan with a little broth, marjoram, and a pinch of salt. Let them soften over medium heat, then add the fresh and dried mushrooms. Stir, sprinkle with flour and pour in the hot oat milk without stopping stirring from avoiding lumps. Sprinkle with the rest of the hot broth and the soaking water of the porcini mushrooms.

Cook the soup for about 20 minutes, then blend it by immersion. Season it with salt, season it with oil and transfer it to the soup plates, where you have distributed the toasted flakes. Garnish with parsley and serve.

2) Spelled and potato soup

Ingredients:
- **250 g of spelled**
- **3 potatoes**
- **1 red onion**
- **1 heart of celery**
- **2 carrots**
- **100 g of peeled tomatoes**
- **extra virgin olive oil**
- **salt and pepper**

Soak the spelled in cold water overnight. The next day, rinse it and cook it in a pot with one and a half liters of salted water for about 20 minutes. Peel the potatoes and onion, peel the carrot and celery. Cut all the vegetables into cubes or small pieces. In an earthenware pot, first brown a fried onion, celery, and carrots with a salt pinch. Just wilted, add the potatoes and tomatoes. Stew on low heat. Halfway through cooking, pour about a liter of boiling water and continue to cook for 20 minutes. Once cooked, pass the vegetables through a vegetable mill and add the boiled spelled. Mix the ingredients and season with salt and pepper. Serve the soup dressed with raw extra virgin olive oil.

3) Carrot soup with almonds

Ingredients:
- **2 potatoes**
- **1 kg of carrots**
- **500 g of fennel**
- **1 stalk of celery**
- **1 onion**
- **150 g of almonds**
- **1 bunch of parsley**
- **2-3 tablespoons of sunflower oil**

Wash the fennel and celery, peel the onion, potatoes, and carrots; cut the prepared vegetables into small pieces and chop the almonds. Collect everything in a pot. Pour enough water to cover the vegetables by about two fingers. Bring to a boil, reduce the heat; cook for about 30 minutes, remove from heat, and work the mixture with the hand blender until creamy. Season with salt and complete with the washed and chopped parsley and sunflower oil.

4)   Pumpkin and cauliflower soup

Ingredients:
- a small pumpkin
- an onion
- half a teaspoon of salt
- a cup of cauliflower
- a teaspoon of white miso

In a saucepan, arrange the diced onion and diced pumpkin. Cover with water, add salt and cook until the vegetables are well softened. Blend until you get a soft pumpkin cream. In a saucepan of boiling water, cook the pieces of cauliflower for 2-3 minutes. Drain and add them to the pumpkin cream. Dress with white miso. Garnish with parsley and serve.

5)   Spelled and bean soup

Ingredients:
- **120 g of beans**
- **150 g of pearl spelled**
- **1-2 tablespoons of extra virgin olive oil**
- **1 small leek**
- **2 celery sticks**
- **1 carrot**
- **1 piece of pumpkin**
- **1 potato**
- **about 2 liters of vegetable broth**
- **1 bunch of herbs (sage, rosemary, bay leaf)**
- **1 pinch of red pepper**
- **a small sprig of chopped parsley**
- **1 teaspoon of salt**

Soak the beans for 12 hours; remove the soaking water, cover abundantly with fresh water, bring to a boil; then cook for an hour and a half over low heat, adding salt towards the end of cooking. Take half of the beans with the cooking water and pass them through a vegetable mill. Cut the vegetables into cubes, toss the leek in the oil first for 1-2 minutes and then all the others with the salt and chilli. Add the spelled, the bunch of herbs and the vegetable broth; cook in a covered pot over low heat for 30 minutes. Add the beans (pureed and whole), and continue cooking for another 15 minutes. Let the soup rest for about an hour before serving (but it is also good right away!), Garnish each portion with a drizzle of oil and chopped parsley.

6)   Cream of barley

Ingredients:
- **300 g of barley**
- **2 l of vegetable broth**
- **1 sprig of rosemary**
- **1 clove of garlic**
- **2 carrots**
- **2 sticks of celery with the leaves**
- **1 onion**
- **1 kohlrabi with leaves**
- **6 sprigs of parsley**
- **4 tablespoons of soy cream**
- **2 teaspoons of turmeric**

Soak the barley overnight, then drain and rinse it. Boil the broth with garlic and rosemary without the sprig. Add the barley, lower the heat and cook for 30 minutes.
Meanwhile, clean the carrots, celery, onion, and kohlrabi. Cut them into small pieces and add them to the barley. Season with turmeric and pepper. Continue cooking for about 20 minutes. Finally, pass everything to the mixer. Add the soy cream and heat the cream over low heat. Season with salt and serve.

7) Colorful buckwheat salad

Ingredients:
- **300 g of buckwheat**
- **2 bay leaves**
- **250 g of boiled green beans**
- **4 ripe tomatoes**
- **1 large bunch of fresh basil**
- **100 g of green olives**
- **1 small clove of garlic**
- **200 g of canned corn**
- **oil**
- **salt and pepper**

Toast the buckwheat without adding fat and cook it with double the water for 20 minutes: when it boils, lower the heat and cook covered with salt and bay leaf. Drain it and let it cool. Meanwhile, wash the tomatoes and green beans, remove the seeds from the first and chop with the second. Rinse the basil well and blend it with the pitted olives, the chopped garlic in quarters, pepper, salt, and oil. Spread the dressing over the cereal, mix the other ingredients and serve this salad cold.

8)   Peach, parmesan and rocket salad

Ingredients:
- **2 yellow peaches**
- **80 g of rocket**
- **80 g parmesan**
- **7-8 tablespoons of extra virgin olive oil**
- **3 teaspoons of black sesame seeds**
- **salt**

Divide the peaches in half, remove the stone and peel them (if they are too ripe, peel them before halving and peeling them); then slice them thinly. Arrange the washed and dried rocket on four plates; distribute the prepared fruits and season the salad with oil and a light sprinkling of salt. Ultimate by distributing in each portion the parmesan reduced to flakes and sesame seeds.

9)   Cold avocado soup

Ingredients:
- **1 handful of fresh coriander**
- **1 clove of garlic**
- **a few tufts of chives**
- **the juice of 1 lime**
- **a few pinches of cumin powder**
- **a few pinches of nutmeg**
- **salt**
- **black pepper**

Combine the peeled and pitted avocados, the peeled and chopped garlic, the cleaned and chopped chives, the lime, the cumin, the nutmeg, salt, and pepper in a blender. Blend, adding cold water in small quantities until you reach a soft consistency. Add the washed and chopped coriander, work the mixture again to mix it, and transfer it to a bowl. Put it in the refrigerator to cool. Serve it in individual bowls, completing, if you like, with a little cream and a few leaves of fresh coriander or chopped chives.

10) Cream of spinach with pine nuts

Ingredients:
- **1 kg of spinach**
- **2 shallots**
- **500 ml of vegetable broth**
- **100 ml of soy milk**
- **100 g of creamy tofu**
- **2 tablespoons of flour**
- **2 tablespoons of pine nuts**
- **2 teaspoons of turmeric**
- **2 tablespoons of oil**
- **salt and pepper**

Clean the spinach, wash and drain them. Finely chop the shallots and let them soften in a saucepan with a little broth for about ten minutes. Add the flour, stir to avoid lumps, and add the spinach. Add salt, stir briefly and pour in the warmed milk and remaining broth, tofu, and turmeric. Cook for about ten minutes and blend by immersion. Peppered, seasoned with oil, and served garnished with lightly toasted pine nuts and, if desired, with oat cakes.

11) Barley and bean soup

Ingredients:
- **200 g of cooked beans**
- **150 g of pearl barley**
- **1 small onion**
- **1 small carrot**
- **1 stalk of celery**
- **100 g approx. of pumpkin pulp**
- **1 sprig of parsley**
- **1 clove of garlic**
- **4 tablespoons of oil**
- **1 pinch of chilli**
- **salt**

Boil the barley in 400 ml of water with a pinch of salt, for about 40 minutes, in a covered pot. Prepare a mixture of garlic, onion, celery, carrot, and parsley; cut the pumpkin into cubes. Fry the mixture in oil in a large pot with a pinch of salt; then add the pumpkin and let it simmer for five minutes, until softened, possibly with a little water. Then add the barley and beans with their cooking water or a little broth to get the right consistency (the soup should be creamy); bring to a boil and cook for another 5 minutes. Season with a pinch of chili and serve hot. Alternatively, you can cook the barley directly with the vegetables and add the beans towards cooking.

12) Spelled with avocado, orange and capers

Ingredients:
- **250 g of peeled spelled**
- **1 small avocado**
- **1 orange**
- **2 small handfuls of salted capers**
- **oil, to taste**
- **the juice of ½ lemon**
- **whole sea salt, to taste**
- **dried oregano, to taste**
- **white pepper, to taste**

Wash the spelled under cold running water and drain it. Cook it for about 45 minutes in filtered water, over low heat and with a lid, using 2 parts of water for one cereal part. Drain it and let it cool. In the meantime, clean the avocado, cut it into small pieces, peel the orange, divide it into raw peeled wedges, and then cut them into small pieces. Soak the capers in filtered water for 10-15 minutes, then rinse and squeeze them well. Add the already cooked spelled, cold or at room temperature, the avocado, the orange, and the capers in a salad bowl. Season with extra virgin olive oil, lemon juice, and salt, add the dried, chopped oregano and freshly ground pepper, and mix well. Serve immediately, or keep the spelled salad in the refrigerator until ready to serve.

Chapter 7: Fish and Seafood

1)   Salad rolls stuffed with tuna

Ingredients:
- **Tuna fillet 100 g**
- **Lettuce 4 leaves**
- **Broad beans 400 g**
- **Extra virgin olive oil 40 g**
- **Basil 3 leaves**
- **Salt up to taste**
- **Low-fat yogurt 20 g**
- **Chopped pistachios to taste**
- **Chives 8 strands**

Shell the beans and collect them in the mixer's glass, pour the olive oil, and blend to obtain a cream. Also, add the yogurt, salt, and mix with a spoon to combine. Scent, the cream with the chopped basil, leaves with your hands. In a pan with a drizzle of oil, brown the tuna for a few minutes. Now take the lettuce leaves, wash them well under running water, then dry them thoroughly with a cloth. Divide each leaf in half, taking care to remove the more rigid central core. Take one half of the lettuce leaf, spread the cream of beans and yogurt, and the entire leaf and stuff with the cooked tuna cut into chunks. Roll up the leaf, tie it with a thread of chives to seal the roll. Garnish with chopped pistachios to taste and continue in the same way for all the others. Your salad rolls stuffed with tuna are ready to be brought to the table. Accompany them with an extra cream of broad beans!

2)   Cod with yogurt and purple potatoes

Ingredients;
- **Cod 400 g**
- **Natural white yogurt 120 g**
- **Purple potatoes 200 g**
- **Extra virgin olive oil 60 g**
- **Salt up to taste**
- **Thyme to taste**
- **4 slices bread**
- **Vegetable butter 40 g**

Take the cod fillets, and boil them in a pot for about 10 minutes, until they are white and tender. Pour the potatoes into cold water and cook for about 15 minutes from boiling. Then drain and peel them. In a blender, pour the cod and purple potatoes, peeled and coarsely cut into pieces, add the extra virgin olive oil, season with salt and start blending everything. Keep running the mixer while adding the white yogurt, then work until you get a smooth and whipped cream. Add the thyme leaves. Transfer the mixture to the fridge for at least 10-15 minutes. Cut 4 slices of bread, then take the butter and spread it on the bread, then arrange them on a dripping pan lined with baking paper and toast the slices in a static oven preheated to 200 ° for about 10 minutes, until they are golden brown. Serve your creamy cod mousse with yogurt and purple potatoes on the toasted bread, and add a few thyme leaves.

3)   Tuna with sesame

Ingredients:
- **Tuna (4 fillets) 150 g**
- **Black sesame seeds 10 g**
- **White sesame seeds 20 g**
- **Extra virgin olive oil 35 g**
- **Lemon juice 25 g**
- **Salt up to taste**

In a dish, pour the sesame seeds, and mix them. Take the tuna: we recommend that you make sure that the tuna you have purchased has been slaughtered; however, we recommend that you freeze it for at least 96 hours at -18 degrees, then defrost it before using the recipe. Pass the slices of tuna over the seeds to bread them on both sides as evenly as possible. Heat a non-stick pan and only when it is hot, place the breaded tuna fillets and cook over high heat for 1 minute, then turn them with a spatula, continue cooking for another minute. Once seared, the tuna will be raw inside, but you can extend the cooking according to your taste if you like. Once cooked, transfer the fillets to a cutting board, immediately cut them into slices, and serve immediately.

4)   Sea bream with carrots and zucchini

Ingredients:
- **Sea bream 2 pieces (clean)**
- **Extra virgin olive oil 30 g**
- **Carrots 150 g**
- **Zucchini 150 g**
- **Thyme to taste**

Wash and peel the carrots, then trim the ends and cut them into slices of about 5 mm thick. Wash and trim the zucchini, too, cut them in half lengthwise and then further divide each half; finally, cut them into cubes of about 1 cm thick. Pour the oil into a large non-stick pan and when it is hot, place the sea bream inside, then add the carrots, the zucchini, the spring onion, and the sprigs of thyme, and add salt. Cover the pan with a lid and cook over medium heat for 7 minutes, then turn the sea bream with the help of 2 spatulas, being careful not to break them; cover again with the lid and cook for another 7 minutes. Of course, cooking times may vary depending on the weight of the sea bream you will use. The pan-fried sea bream is ready to be served!

5) Swordfish and broccoli medallions

Ingredients:
- **Swordfish fillet 400 g**
- **Broccoli 200 g**
- **Potatoes 400 g**
- **Marjoram 3 sprigs**
- **Extra virgin olive oil q.s.**
- **Salt up to taste**

Put two pans with water to bring to the boil; in one place, the thoroughly washed potatoes when the water is still cold, when it boils, calculate for about 30-40 minutes. Meanwhile, wash the broccoli, put them in the other pan when the water has boiled, and simmer for about 5 minutes. Then drain the broccoli and chop coarsely with a knife, then let them cool. When the potatoes are cooked, peel and mash them with a potato masher in a large bowl, then preheat the oven to 200 ° in static mode. Finally, take the swordfish fillets, cut them into cubes, and then chop them coarsely with a knife. When the vegetables have cooled, take the bowl where you mashed the potatoes, add the chopped broccoli and swordfish, salt, and add the marjoram leaves, then mix with your hands to mix all the ingredients. Take some dough and shape it with a 6.5 cm diameter pastry ring to form the medallions: with these doses, you should get 6. Transfer the medallions on a baking tray lined with parchment paper, season with a drizzle of oil, then bake them in a preheated static oven at 200 ° for about 20 minutes.

After the medallions' cooking time, take them out of the oven and transfer them to a serving dish, add a few leaves of marjoram, and season with a drizzle of raw oil. Your cod and broccoli medallions are ready to be served!

6)   Cod fillet with pistachio pesto

Ingredients:
- **Cod fillets 2**
- **Extra virgin olive oil q.s.**
- **Salt up to taste**

FOR THE PISTACHIO PESTO
- **Unsalted pistachios 30 g**
- **Extra virgin olive oil 30 g**
- **Salt up to taste**

Pour the shelled pistachios into a blender, add the oil and a pinch of salt, and blend until a smooth cream is obtained, then transfer the pistachio pesto into a bowl and set aside. Heat a little oil in a non-stick pan, add the cod fillets, add salt and cook over medium-high heat for 2-3 minutes. At this point, gently turn the fillets with a spatula and cook them on the other side for 1-2 minutes, then remove them from the pan. Spread a spoonful of pistachio pesto on each plate, place the cod fillet. Your cod fillet with pistachio pesto is ready to serve!

7)   Shrimp with dried tomatoes

Ingredients:
- **Shelled and cleaned shrimp 500 g**
- **Anchovies 6**
- **Dried tomatoes 6**
- **A handful of capers**
- **Tomatoes 4**
- **Garlic cloves 3**
- **Pitted olives 10**
- **Lemon 1**
- **Black pepper to taste**
- **Parsley to taste**
- **Basil to taste**

Heat olive oil over medium-high heat in a large pan. Add the prawns, peeled and cleaned, with half a teaspoon of salt and half of black pepper; cook for 5 minutes, occasionally turning the prawns. Put the prawns in a bowl and keep them warm. Pour the wine into the pan, mix, and let it evaporate. Cut the fresh and dried tomatoes, add the garlic and cook in a pan over medium heat until everything is softened (about 3 minutes). Take the lemon, cut the peel and chop it, add the shredded anchovies, two tablespoons of capers, parsley olives, and basil. Cook for 2 minutes, mixing everything. Return the prawns to the pan and mix. Serve immediately.

8)   Baked sea bream

Ingredients:
- **Sea bream 2 cleaned**
- **Garlic 1 clove**
- **Salt to taste**
- **Black pepper to taste**
- **Parsley 2 tufts**
- **Thyme 2 sprigs**
- **Extra virgin olive oil 20 g**
- **Lemons 1 slice**

Preheat the oven to 180C. Wash and chop the parsley. Place a parchment paper sheet on a baking tray and place each clean sea bream in the center, salt, and pepper the inside. Then stuffed with the aromas: sprigs of thyme previously washed and dried, half a clove of peeled garlic for each sea bream, half a slice of lemon, and extra virgin olive oil. Pour in a drizzle of olive oil also over the sea bream, close the parchment paper sheet by rolling the two ends. Then wrap it in aluminum foil, wrinkling the ends in this case too to seal. Place the sea bream on a baking sheet and bake in a preheated static oven at 180 ° for about 40 minutes. When cooked, take the sea bream out of the oven, let it cool and then serve it in the same foil, sprinkling it with fresh parsley if you like.

9) Baked sea bream

Ingredients:

- **Sea bream 2 cleaned**
- **Garlic 1 clove**
- **Salt to taste**
- **Black pepper to taste**
- **Parsley 2 tufts**
- **Thyme 2 sprigs**
- **Extra virgin olive oil 20 g**
- **Lemons 1 slice**

Preheat the oven to 180C. Wash and chop the parsley. Place a parchment paper sheet on a baking tray and place each clean sea bream in the center, salt, and pepper the inside. Then stuffed with the aromas: sprigs of thyme previously washed and dried, half a clove of peeled garlic for each sea bream, half a slice of lemon, and extra virgin olive oil. Pour in a drizzle of olive oil also over the sea bream, close the parchment paper sheet by rolling the two ends. Then wrap it in aluminum foil, wrinkling the ends in this case too to seal. Place the sea bream on a baking sheet and bake in a preheated static oven at 180 ° for about 40 minutes. When cooked, take the sea bream out of the oven, let it cool and then serve it in the same foil, sprinkling it with fresh parsley if you like.

10) Salmon rice

Ingredients:
- **Rice 350 g**
- **Salmon steaks 250 g**
- **Leeks 1**
- **Extra virgin olive oil q.s.**
- **1 clove garlic**
- **½ glass white wine**
- **Parmesan to be grated 20 g**
- **Salt up to taste**
- **Black pepper to taste**
- **Fish broth 500 ml**

FOR THE FLAVORED BUTTER
- **Butter 80 g**
- **Marjoram 1 sprig**
- **Dill 1 sprig**
- **Thyme 1 sprig**
- **Lemon zest ½**
- **Salt up to taste**

Prepare the flavored butter by chopping the herbs and grating the lemon zest, allow the butter to soften at room temperature and when it has reached a creamy consistency add the chopped herbs, lemon zest and salt. Meanwhile, clean the salmon steak and cut it into small pieces. Heat a tablespoon of oil in a pan with a clove of whole garlic and brown the salmon bites for 2/3 minutes, add salt and set the salmon aside, removing the garlic. Now start preparing the risotto: finely chop the leek and sauté it over low heat with two tablespoons of oil in a pan.

Pour in the rice and toast it for a few moments over high heat, stirring with a wooden spoon. Deglaze with the counter wine and continue cooking, stirring occasionally, taking care that the rice does not stick, adding the broth (vegetable or fish) a little at a time. Halfway through cooking add the salmon morsels, season with salt if necessary and when the rice is well cooked, remove it from the heat and stir in the herb-flavored butter and a couple of tablespoons of grated cheese, if you like.

11) Crispy salmon

Ingredients:
- **Salmon fillet (4 of 250 g each) 1 kg**
- **Bread 100 g**
- **1 sprig parsley**
- **Dill 1 sprig**
- **Thyme 4 sprigs**
- **Rosemary 2 sprigs**
- **Lemon zest 1**
- **Extra virgin olive oil 50 g**
- **White pepper in grains 1 tsp**
- **Salt up to taste**

First, prepare the breading: cut the bread into pieces and put it in a mixer, then add the dill, the peeled thyme, the needles of rosemary and parsley. Pour in the oil too, then add the lemon zest, salt and white pepper. Blend until you get a coarse consistency. Now take care of the salmon fillets: remove the skin with a thin-bladed knife and remove the bones with the help of a kitchen tongs, then transfer the fillets to a drip pan lined with parchment paper and cover them with the breading, making it adhere well with your hands. . After covering the fillets evenly, cook in a preheated convection oven at 190 ° for about 20 minutes. After the cooking time, take out and serve your crispy salmon hot!

12) Baked sardines

Ingredients:
- **18 sardines for a total of about 250 g**
- **Breadcrumbs 60 g**
- **Extra virgin olive oil 60 g**
- **1 sprig parsley**
- **Thyme 1 sprig**
- **1 clove garlic**
- **Grated Parmesan cheese 20 g**
- **Pine nuts 30 g**
- **Extra virgin olive oil to grease the pan 15g**

Pour the breadcrumbs, grated cheese and the crushed garlic clove into a bowl. Rinse, dry and finely chop the parsley; then also add it to the breading and further flavor with the thyme leaves; pour the 60 g of oil and mix everything until you get a uniform mixture. At this point take a baking dish measuring 19x15 cm and sprinkle it with about 15 g of oil. Arrange the sardines horizontally without overlapping each other, salt (not excessively), pepper and cover with half of the previously prepared mixture. Arrange another layer of sardines, taking care to position them vertically (opposite to before), salt, pepper and cover the entire surface with the remaining part of the breading. Finish by decorating the surface with pine nuts. Then cook the sardines in the oven in grill mode at 200 ° for 8 minutes, until they are golden brown. Once cooked, serve the baked sardines while still hot.

Chapter 8: Meat

1) Chunks of chicken in fennel sauce

Ingredients:
- **Chicken breasts g 600**
- **Fennel n 3 medium**
- **Garlic cloves 2**
- **Dry oregano 1/2 tsp**
- **Chili powder 1/4 tsp**
- **Chopped onion 4 tbsp**
- **Extra virgin olive oil**
- **Salt and pepper**

In a large skillet, heat the oil and quickly brown the diced chicken over high heat. Brown on all sides, then drain and keep warm. In the same pan, add the chopped onion, garlic, and cook over low heat for a few minutes. Add the cleaned, washed, and thinly sliced fennel. Wet with two water glasses, add the salt, chili pepper, and oregano, cover, and simmer for about 20 minutes or until the water has dried, and the fennel is almost reduced to cream. Bring the chicken back on the heat, stir, and cook for another 5 minutes. Turn off and serve hot.

2) Roast turkey stuffed with broccoli

Ingredients:
- **Turkey breast 700 g**
- **Broccoli tops 250 g**
- **1 egg white**
- **Garlic 1 clove**
- **1 pinch chili**
- **2 tablespoons olive oil**
- **Salt to taste**

Preheat the oven to 180C. In a pot filled with salted water, boil the broccoli until tender. Drain just ready. In a pan heat 1 tablespoon of oil and brown the minced garlic for a few minutes. Add the tops of boiled broccoli and the chili pepper. Cook for a few minutes, until they are well flavored. Turn off and let cool, then add the egg white and mix well. On the cutting board, roll out the turkey breast, cut a side pocket, and stuff with broccoli. Close with kitchen string, brush with the rest of the oil and inform at 180 ° for 40 minutes. Turn once. If necessary, moisten with a little broth. Remove from the oven and leave to rest for a few minutes, then slice and serve hot.

3) Baked lamb chops

Ingredients:
- **Lamb chops 800 g**
- **Thyme 2 sprigs**
- **Rosemary 3 sprigs**
- **Salt to taste**
- **Black peppercorns to taste**
- **2 cloves garlic**
- **Extra virgin olive oil 40 g**
- **Lemon zest 1**
- **Black pepper to taste**

Start cleaning the meat from excess fat, then make cuts between one rib and the other and, with the help of your fingers, push the meat down to free the bone as much as possible. Transfer the ribs to an ovenproof dish and season with 4 salt and pepper. Also, add 2 sprigs of rosemary, thyme, and peppercorns. Pour about 10 g of oil, add the freshly grated lemon zest, and sprinkle all the ribs. Also, add a clove of garlic divided in half, cover with plastic wrap, and leave to marinate for about 2 hours in the refrigerator. Place the ribs on a lightly greased baking dish. Wrap the bones with a strip of aluminum foil, completely cover them and not let them burn during cooking. Then bake in a preheated static oven at 200 ° for 50 minutes. Once cooked, take out of the oven and serve your lamb chops in the oven.

4)   Turkey burger

Ingredients:
- **Wholemeal hamburger buns 4**
- **Ground turkey 600 g**
- **Aubergines 480 g**
- **Auburn tomatoes 320 g**
- **Green salad 60 g**
- **Rosemary to taste**
- **Oregano to taste**
- **Thyme to taste**
- **Salt to taste**
- **Black pepper to taste**
- **Extra virgin olive oil 10 g**

Start by chopping the aromatic herbs: rosemary, oregano, and thyme. In a bowl, add the minced meat with the mince; season with salt and pepper. Knead all the ingredients by hand and let the mixture rest in the refrigerator for 15 minutes. Meanwhile, wash and tick the aubergine removing the ends. Slice it about half a centimeter thick and place it on a well-heated and lightly greased plate. After a few minutes of cooking, turn the aubergine discs so you will also cook them on the other side at the end of cooking, set aside. Browse your salad and rinse it thoroughly to get rid of soil residues, then transfer the lettuce onto a tray with paper towels and gently dab it to dry; in this way, you will not damage it. Finally, wash the tomato and slice it in half centimeter thick slices after having stripped it of the stalk. At this point, all your ingredients are ready.

Take the minced meat from the fridge and place it inside
an 11 cm circular pasta bowl that you will have placed on
a parchment paper sheet. Then help yourself with the
back of a spoon to level the surface to smooth and brush
each hamburger with a little oil.

Place the meat medallions on the hot grill, and after 4
minutes of cooking, you can turn them with the help of a
spatula to cook them on the other side for the same time.
If you want a well-warmed and slightly toasted sandwich,
cut the bread into two parts, then arrange the two parts
on the still hot grill, letting go for a few minutes, until the
base has become crispy.

As soon as your sandwiches are hot, switch to the
composition: then on the sandwich base lay 3-4 lettuce
leaves and 4 tomato disks, then 4 slices of aubergines and
finally your meat medallion. Close with the other half of
bread, and your turkey burgers are ready to be bitten still
hot!

5)   Chicken and green beans rolls

Ingredients:

- **Chicken breast (8 slices of 30g) 240g**
- **Fresh green beans 100 g**
- **Raw ham (8 slices) 70 g**
- **Salt up to taste**
- **Extra virgin olive oil 15 g**

FOR THE YOGURT POTATO SALAD

- **Potatoes 500 g**
- **White yogurt 100 g**
- **Partially skimmed milk 20 g**
- **Chives 3 strands**
- **Salt up to taste**
- **Black pepper to taste**

Pour the potatoes into a saucepan with plenty of cold water, place it on the stove and let it boil, then cook the potatoes for 20-30 minutes depending on their size, doing a test with a fork. The potatoes will be cooked as soon as they no longer resist, at which point drain them and let them cool a little, then peel them and let them cool. Once the boiled potatoes are completely cooled, cut them into pieces of a couple of centimeters. Collect the cubes in a container and pour the yogurt together with the chives that you can cut with scissors and mix. If you notice that the mixture becomes too thick, dissolve by adding 1-2 tablespoons of milk, season with salt and pepper, mix, and place in the refrigerator, covering with cling film.

Meanwhile, tick the green beans, then remove the two ends, rinse them under running water and blanch them in plenty of boiling water for 10-15 minutes. Then drain the green beans and let them cool a little, adding a little cold water to stop cooking, so they will remain a nice green color. Finally, arrange the green beans in a bowl and season with salt. Arrange the slices of chicken breast on a cutting board and salt them only on the surface. Just above the center, place a handful of green beans. Starting from the highest part, roll the chicken slice with the green beans in the middle to roll up the meat on itself and thus obtain a roll; repeat the operation for all the other slices. Insert two toothpicks for each roll; in this way, you will be sure that it does not open during cooking. Pour extra virgin olive oil into a pan and when it is hot, place the rolls, turning them over after a few minutes of cooking over high heat and continue to seal the meat well. Let them cool for a few moments, and do not throw away the cooking oil that will be used later. Remove the wooden skewers from each roll and salt the surface that was not previously salted. Arrange the slices of raw ham on a cutting board and starting from the bottom roll the slice all around the roll so that the ham completely covers the roll and does so for everyone. In a baking dish, pour the rolls' cooking juices and place them in them, letting them cook in a static oven preheated to 180 ° for 15 minutes. As soon as the chicken and green bean rolls are cooked, you can serve them with your yogurt potato salad!

6)   Turkey steak with fennel and pomegranate

Ingredients:
- **Whole turkey breast 800 g**
- **Fennel 400 g**
- **Pomegranate (1 medium) 400 g**
- **Extra virgin olive oil 80 g**
- **Black pepper to taste**
- **Salt up to taste**
- **Dill to taste**
- **Salt to taste**

On a hot plate, pour a drizzle of oil. Place the turkey on it and cook over medium heat on the first side for about 25 minutes. After the first 25 minutes, turn it over and cook for another 25 on the other side. In the meantime, prepare the dressing: take the pomegranate, cut it in half and shell it, collecting the beans in a bowl; keep some aside for the final decoration, pour the others into a mixer, and blend. Then pass the puree obtained through a colander to filter the juice you can put in a tall glass. Add 40 g of oil, salt, and pepper. Blend everything. Wash and trim the fennel to remove the green part. Divide it in half, then slice it finely, then transfer it to a bowl to the season with 30 g of oil, salt, and pepper. Flavor with the chopped dill with your hands. Stir and spread on a serving dish. Take the turkey, cut it to a thickness of about 1 cm for each slice, and distribute it on the bed of fennel. Season with the pomegranate seeds kept aside sprinkle with the pomegranate and oil emulsion; your sliced turkey with fennel and pomegranate is ready to be served.

7) Baked chicken legs with apples

Ingredients:
- **Chicken legs (4 spindles) 500 g**
- **White wine 50 g**
- **Extra virgin olive oil 40 g**
- **Salt up to 10 g**
- **Sweet paprika to taste**
- **Black pepper in grains to taste**
- **Pink peppercorns to taste**
- **White pepper in grains to taste**
- **Juniper berries to taste**
- **Parsley to taste**
- **Sage as needed**
- **Rosemary to taste**
- **Thyme to taste**

FOR APPLES
- **Fuji apples (about 2) 500 g**
- **Brown sugar 5 g**
- **Salt up to 5 g**
- **Water 50 g**
- **½ lemon juice**

Start by finely chopping the parsley, sage, rosemary, and thyme, and set aside. Put the black, white, and pink peppercorns and juniper berries in a mortar and press them with the pestle to reduce them to powder. Put the chopped herbs and ground spices in a jug, pour the olive oil, add 10 g of fine salt, the wine, and flavor with sweet paprika, then mix with a spoon to flavor. Take an ovenproof dish and grease the bottom with olive oil, place your chicken thighs next to each other here, then cover them with the previously prepared minced spice. Cook the legs in a preheated static oven at 180 ° for 45 minutes. In the meantime, wash and dry the apples, cut them first in half and then into quarters, and finally cut them into smaller and irregular pieces. Pour the apple pieces into a pan, add the brown sugar, 5 g of fine salt, and sprinkle with half a lemon juice. Cook over medium heat to dissolve the sugar, then pour in the water, lower the heat and continue cooking for 10 minutes until the apples are soft. Meanwhile, even the chicken will have finished cooking and will be golden on the surface, so take out and immediately serve your chicken legs in the oven with apples!

8)   Turkey breast with raw ham

Ingredients:

- **Turkey breast 1.2 kg**
- **Sliced raw ham 150 g**
- **White wine 300 ml**
- **Vegetable broth 250 ml**
- **Extra virgin olive oil 30 ml**
- **00 flour 3 tbsp**
- **Rosemary to taste**
- **Sage as needed**
- **Salt up to ½ tsp**

First, lightly salt the meat and massage it. Take the slices of ham and place them on top of the turkey breast. At this point, take care of tying the roast with kitchen twine. Insert a few sprigs of rosemary between the kitchen string. Pour the extra virgin olive oil into a large pan and. Place the stuffed turkey breast, a few sprigs of rosemary, and the sage leaves on top. Let it brown over medium heat for about 5 minutes, turn it over and let it brown on the other side for another 5 minutes. Pour 200 ml of white wine into the pan and after 5 minutes also the vegetable broth. Cover with a lid and let the roast cook over medium heat for about 50 minutes. Preheat the oven to 170 degrees. Transfer the roast to a baking dish and leave it to warm in the oven for 10 minutes. Strain the cooking juices left in the pan and transfer it to a saucepan. Add the remaining 100 ml of white wine and the flour. Mix well and let the sauce thicken over low heat, stirring with a whisk for 4-5 minutes. Gently remove the string by cutting it into several parts with scissors. Slice the turkey breast and serve with the sauce.

9) Chicken with tomatoes and avocado

Ingredients:
- **Chicken breast 550 g**
- **Extra virgin olive oil as needed**
- **Salt up to 1**
- **Black pepper 1 tsp**
- **Lime 1**
- **Oregano 1 tsp**

FOR THE SIDE
- **Copper tomatoes 500 g**
- **Avocado 200 g**
- **Red onions 100 g**
- **Salt up to 1 tsp**
- **Paprika 1 tsp**
- **Black pepper 1 tsp**

First, cut the chicken breast into slices, beat them with a meat mallet to make them thinner. Transfer the meat to a pan, then season with oil, salt, and pepper. Also, add the lime zest and its juice, finally flavored with oregano. Mix well to flavor. Cover with cling film and set aside until ready for cooking. Now take care of the tomatoes: after having washed and dried them, cut them into wedges, and then cut them into cubes. Peel and chop the red onion. In a bowl, combine the tomatoes and onion. Now divide the avocado in half, cut the pulp vertically, and then horizontally to obtain cubes. Pour the avocado into the bowl. Season with oil, paprika, salt, and pepper. Now go to cooking: heat a grill well, place the chicken breasts, and cook for 5 minutes.

Then turn them and continue cooking for another 5 minutes. Once cooked, immediately serve the chicken with the diced tomatoes and avocado.

10) Roasted rabbit

Ingredients:
- **Rabbit in pieces 1.2 kg**
- **Rosemary 4 sprigs**
- **Salt up to taste**
- **Black pepper to taste**
- **Vegetable broth 150 g**
- **Potatoes 800 g**
- **Red onions 120 g**
- **Thyme 4 sprigs**
- **White wine 40 g**
- **1 clove garlic**
- **Bay leaf 1 leaf**
- **Extra virgin olive oil 70 g**

Chop the rosemary, then transfer half of it into a pan where you have poured 40 g of oil and add the peeled clove of garlic. Add a bay leaf and let it cook over low heat for 2-3 minutes. At this point, raise the heat and add the pieces of rabbit, let them brown on both sides for 3-4 minutes, add salt and pepper and blend with the white wine. Once the alcoholic part has evaporated, add a ladle of broth and cook over low heat for another 5-6 minutes. Meanwhile, prepare the potatoes, peel them, and cut them into rather large chunks. Also, cut the onion into slices and transfer everything to a bowl flavored with the rosemary needles, the thyme leaves, salt, and pepper. Drizzle with 20 g of oil and mix potatoes and onions to make them flavor evenly. Transfer everything to a large pan, oiled with about 10 g of oil. Arrange the previously browned rabbit pieces, potatoes, and onions. Add the remaining vegetable broth and cook the rabbit with the potatoes in a preheated static oven at 200 ° for 40 minutes. Once out of the oven, serve your rabbit in the oven while still steaming!

11) Baked meatballs

Ingredients:

- **Minced veal 400 g**
- **1 clove garlic**
- **Stale bread 100 g**
- **Parmesan to grate 100 g**
- **Eggs 2**
- **1 sprig parsley**
- **Salt up to taste**
- **Black pepper to taste**
- **Extra virgin olive oil 2 tbsp**

Start by placing the ground beef in a large bowl, then add the finely chopped stale bread crumbs, the grated cheese, and the chopped parsley and garlic. Finally, add the eggs, season with salt and pepper to taste. Mix the mixture well with a wooden spoon so that all the ingredients are well blended. Cover with cling film and let it rest in the refrigerator for at least half an hour. After this time, form lightly crushed meatballs of the size you prefer with your hands. Lightly oil an ovenproof dish and place the meatballs on it. Add a drizzle of oil and bake in a preheated static oven at 180 ° C for about 40 minutes, until the surface is golden brown. Serve the baked meatballs hot!

12) Chicken legs in yogurt

Ingredients:
- **Chicken thighs 4**
- **Natural white yogurt 250 g**
- **Partially screamed milk 60 g**
- **Extra virgin olive oil 20 g**
- **2 cloves garlic**
- **Oregano to taste**
- **Salt up to taste**

FOR THE ACCOMPANYING SAUCE
- **Natural white yogurt 100 g**
- **Extra virgin olive oil 5 g**
- **½ lemon juice**
- **Lemon zest 1**
- **Salt up to taste**

Pour the yogurt, milk, olive oil, and peeled garlic cloves into the glass of a blender and blend until you get a smooth sauce, then add salt and flavored with oregano, mix everything to flavor. Now place the chicken legs side by side in a large bowl, cover the meat with the yogurt-based marinade, turn them over to moisten completely. Wrap the bowl with cling film and place in the refrigerator to marinate for at least 30 minutes. After the resting time has elapsed, heat a drizzle of olive oil in a pan, place the thighs, and cover them with the yogurt marinade. Cook the chicken over medium heat for about 10 minutes. Once the pan's cooking time has elapsed, transfer the chicken to a baking sheet, season with a drizzle of olive oil and a teaspoon of oregano. Cook the chicken in a preheated static oven at 220 ° for about 20 minutes. While the chicken is cooking in the oven, take care of the accompanying sauce: pour the yogurt into a bowl, add the lemon juice, the oil, a pinch of salt, and flavor with the lemon zest. Stir in the sauce to flavor it. In the meantime, the chicken will be cooked, take it out of the oven and serve the chicken legs in yogurt with the flavored lemon sauce.

Chapter 9: Single course

1) Lentil and rice pie

Ingredients:
- **200 g of lentils**
- **250 g of rice**
- **vegetable broth**
- **2 shallots**
- **2 carrots**
- **1 medium potato**
- **500 g of celeriac**
- **1 bay leaf**
- **3 tablespoons of oil**
- **2 tablespoons of tamari**
- **bread crumbs**
- **3 tablespoons of sesame**
- **1 teaspoon of paprika**
- **1 teaspoon of oregano**
- **salt and chilli**

Soak the lentils for a few hours, drain and boil them for about 40 minutes in water with the bay leaf. Salt towards the end. Gather the rice and 600 ml of broth in a saucepan. With the lid on, boil and reduce the heat. Cook until the liquid runs out. Finely chop the shallots and place them in a pan with oregano, chili, and paprika. Salt and add enough water to cover flush. Cook over medium heat, stirring occasionally. After a few minutes, add the potato, carrots, and celeriac cut into cubes. Stir and pour in a little hot broth. Stew over low heat, adding more hot broth when needed. In the end, transfer the vegetables to the mixer to obtain a thick and creamy mixture, helping you in the case with a little broth. Grease a mold with a bit of oil where you transfer the rice mixed with the lentils. Drizzle with the remaining oil and soy sauce. Cover with vegetable cream and sprinkle with breadcrumbs mixed with sesame. Bake at 180 degrees for about 20 minutes. Serve the pie hot.

2)   Ricotta and walnut pie

Ingredients:
- **500 g of ricotta**
- **4-5 tablespoons of lightly toasted walnuts**
- **2 tablespoons of milk**
- **4 nice pinches of saffron stigmas**
- **3 tablespoons of marjoram leaves**
- **salt**
- **oil for the molds**

Infuse the saffron in hot milk for about an hour. Pour the infusion over the ricotta you have sifted into a bowl, add the coarsely chopped walnuts and marjoram, season with salt. Mix all the ingredients to form a cream that you will distribute in the individual round casseroles about 10-12 centimeters wide, greased with a drizzle of oil. Bake for 20 minutes at 180 degrees. When the patties are ready, take them out of the oven and gently remove them from the molds; arrange them in the center of the plates, accompanying them with salads arranged in a crown and possibly dressed with a light vinaigrette.

3)   White bean paté with caper pesto

Ingredients:
- **300 g cannellini beans (cooked weight)**
- **30 g of onion**
- **30 g of Evo oil**
- **20 g of salted capers**
- **15 g of lemon juice**
- **10 g of lemon zest**
- **a bay leaf**

Boil the beans, which you have previously soaked for at least 12 hours, with a bay leaf. Soak the capers in plenty of warm water and leave them to desalt for the entire preparation time. Then reduce them to a puree, mashing them with a fork or blending them with a hand blender. Help yourself with half the oil and lemon juice to make the pate more homogeneous and fluffy. Separately, chop the onion and cut the lemon zest into thin strips. Drain the capers and chop them coarsely. Place the pate on a plate, season it with the remaining extra virgin olive oil, onion, lemon peel, and capers. Serve at the table cold or room temperature, accompanied by slices of toasted bread.

4) Pasta and cauliflower

Ingredients:
- **350 g of wholemeal short pasta**
- **1 cauliflower of 800 g**
- **400 g of peeled tomatoes**
- **3 tablespoons of oil**
- **2 cloves of garlic**
- **1 teaspoon of marjoram**
- **1 teaspoon of spicy paprika**
- **50 g of Parmesan cheese**

Clean the cauliflower, wash it, divide it into florets and steam it for 10-15 minutes. Meanwhile, put the crushed tomatoes with a fork, chopped garlic, marjoram, paprika, salt in a saucepan. Cook them for about 15 minutes. Add the cauliflower. Cook for a few minutes, stirring. Bring water to boil in a saucepan. When it comes to the boil, cook the pasta for the time indicated on the package. Drain and pour the cauliflower pasta. Grate the cheese, turn the heat back on under the pasta and stir for 1 minute over medium heat. Season with oil, season with salt, and serve.

5) Rice salad in tomatoes

Ingredients:
- **4 large ripe but firm tomatoes**
- **200 g of brown rice**
- **500 ml of broth**
- **1 spring onion**
- **80 g of mayonnaise)**
- **10 pitted green olives**
- **a few sprigs of fresh marjoram**
- **salt**

Pour the rice and broth into a saucepan. Put the lid on; when it boils, lower the heat and cook for 40-45 minutes. In the last 10 minutes add the green part of the onion, washed and shredded. When cooked, add salt to the rice and let it cool. Wash the tomatoes, remove the top cap, empty them internally and add salt. Mix the mayonnaise with the rice; if the mixture is too dry, add a little tomato pulp (saving the rest for a salad or a sauce). Incorporate a mixture made with the white onion and marjoram. Complete with the chopped olives and stuff the tomatoes with the mixture obtained. Cover them with the cap and let them rest in the fridge for half an hour before serving.

6)   Pasta with cherry tomatoes and capers

Ingredients:
- **280 g of wholemeal pasta of your choice**
- **12-15 cherry tomatoes, cleaned and quartered**
- **4-5 tablespoons of extra virgin olive oil**
- **half a white onion, peeled and chopped**
- **2 spicy green peppers, cleaned and chopped**
- **1 generous handful of salted capers**
- **1 handful of fresh, clean oregano**

Soak the capers in cold water for about 20 minutes, rinse and drain. Cook the pasta in abundant salted water. Meanwhile, heat the oil in a large pan and lightly soften the onion. Add the chilies, tomatoes and cook the capers for 4-5 minutes beforehand. Once the pasta is cooked, drain and add it to the sauce. Stir a couple of minutes, remove from heat, stir and serve.

7)   Zucchini stuffed with chickpeas

Ingredients:
- **4 medium-large zucchini**
- **vegetable broth q.s.**
- **250 g of boiled chickpeas**
- **2 shallots**
- **1 teaspoon of coriander seeds**
- **20 g of dried mushrooms**
- **1 teaspoon of marjoram**
- **the juice of 1/2 lemon**
- **3 tablespoons of oil**
- **Salt to taste**

Soak the mushrooms in warm water for 30 minutes.
Wash the zucchini and steam them whole for 5 minutes.
Let them cool, tick them, and cut them in half lengthwise;
gently dig them to remove most of the pulp, taking care
not to break the peel. Set them aside. Finely chop the
shallots and let them soften for a few minutes in a pan,
lightly covered with broth. Add the marjoram and the
squeezed and thinly sliced mushrooms. Follow with the
crushed coriander and salt. Cook for 10 minutes on low
heat, finally adds the chickpeas, a tablespoon of oil, and
lemon juice. Stir and turn off the heat. Blend by
immersion, helping you if needed with a little broth but
trying to keep the mixture firm. Transfer it to the zucchini
shells, which you will then line up on a baking sheet lined
with baking paper. Bake at 180 degrees for about 30
minutes. Serve the dish hot or warm, seasoned with the
remaining oil.

8)   Rice and peas

Ingredients:
- **200 g of rice**
- **1 Kg of peas**
- **garlic**
- **parsley**
- **extra virgin olive oil**
- **salt and pepper**

Bring salted water to a boil for cooking the rice.
Meanwhile, in a pan, cook the shelled peas cold with
finely chopped garlic and parsley and a glass of water.
When almost cooked, evaporate any excess water, add
salt, and season with extra virgin olive oil. Serve the
boiled rice with the peas.

9)   Spaghetti with walnut and basil sauce

Ingredients:
- **400 g of spaghetti**
- **100 g of shelled walnuts**
- **80 g of pine nuts**
- **1 clove of garlic**
- **30 g of basil leaves**
- **2 tablespoons of grated parmesan**
- **3 tablespoons of oil**
- **salt**

Prepare the sauce. Spread the walnuts and half of the pine nuts on a baking tray in a single layer. Bake them at 150 ° for about ten minutes until they are lightly toasted. During this time, stir them a couple of times. Let them cool down and remove the skin by rubbing them. Put them in a mixer with a little salt and chop finely. Add the peeled and chopped garlic, then washed and dried basil, a few tablespoons of hot water. Continue to work the ingredients until they are homogeneous, adding a little more hot water. Complete with oil. Cook the spaghetti in boiling salted water, drain when al dente, and season immediately with the walnut and basil sauce. Sprinkle them with the grated Parmesan and serve.

10) Artichoke and lentil cake pan

Ingredients:
- **12 artichokes**
- **1 lemon**
- **300 g of lentils**
- **2 shallots**
- **1 sprig of rosemary**
- **1 sprig of sage**
- **1 teaspoon of thyme**
- **vegetable broth**
- **bread crumbs**
- **4 tablespoons of oil**
- **salt**

Soak the lentils overnight, rinse them and place them in a saucepan with the chopped rosemary and sage. Cover them with cold water and cook for about 40 minutes. Add salt only at the end. Clean the artichokes, halve them and wash them in water acidulated with lemon juice. Cook them al dente in a pan with the thyme, a tablespoon of oil, and a little water, salt. Be careful not to break them and keep them crunchy. Blend the lentils until the mixture is not too moist. Finely chop the shallots, let them dry in a pan with a tablespoon of oil and a little water. Add the past and let it flavor for a few minutes. Add another tablespoon of oil and stir. Grease a round mold with high sides, and sprinkle it with breadcrumbs. Form the first layer with half of the artichokes. Pour half of the remaining oil, distribute the legume purée and arrange the rest of the artichokes on the surface. Season with the remaining oil and bake at 190 ° for 10 minutes. Serve the dish hot.

11) Radicchio and pear risotto with spices

Ingredients:
- **320 g of brown rice**
- **250 g of radicchio**
- **200 g of pears**
- **a few walnut kernels**
- **oil**
- **1 l of vegetable broth**
- **½ glass of white wine**
- **3 cloves**
- **the juice of ½ lemon**
- **salt**

Cut the pears into cubes and sprinkle them with lemon so that they do not darken. Reduce the radicchio (except four or five leaves) into thin strips. Sauté the radicchio with the cloves in a saucepan with some olive oil for a few minutes, add the pears and cook for another minute. Transfer everything to a bowl. Clean the pan's cooking bottom, pour a couple of tablespoons of oil, and toast the washed and drained rice. Deglaze with the wine, season over high heat for one minute. Add the boiling broth a little at a time, waiting for it to be absorbed before adding more. Halfway through cooking, add the radicchio and cooked pears; season with salt. Serve the risotto in the wave, and garnish it with the walnut kernels and raw radicchio leaves.

12) Pumpkin rice

Ingredients:
- **1 cup of brown rice**
- **1 onion**
- **400 g of clean pumpkin**
- **3 cups of vegetable broth**
- **1 sprig of rosemary**
- **3 tablespoons of oil**

Put the rice in a saucepan with 2 cups of broth. Cover and bring it to a boil, then lower the heat and cook slowly for an hour. Meanwhile, finely chop the onion and transfer it to a pan just covered with broth. Let it soften over medium heat for a few minutes before adding the diced pumpkin and rosemary leaves. Pour in the remaining broth and cook over low heat for 10-15 minutes. Add the pumpkin to the cooked rice and leave to rest for 5 minutes. Season with oil and salt, stir, and serve.

Chapter 10: Dessert

1) Buckwheat and dark chocolate cake

Ingredients:
- **100 g dates**
- **200 g buckwheat**
- **60 g bitter cocoa**
- **90 g 95% dark chocolate**
- **Grated orange peel to taste**
- **140 g tofu**
- **½ teaspoon of agar agar**

Soak the buckwheat for 24 hours, then drain and place in a sprouter. Rinse twice a day for 2-3 days, and as soon as it begins to sprout, place in the dryer basket at 42 ° for 8 hours. Blend the sprouted and dried buckwheat, dates, vanilla, and grated orange zest at maximum power. Add the tofu and continue blending. Separately, dissolve the agar agar in cold water and add to the mixture, mixing again. Add the dark chocolate in pieces and bring to a boil for a few minutes. Pour the mixture into a square shape, a level well, and store in the freezer for 3 hours. When the cake is ready, sprinkle with cocoa. Let it rest out of the freezer for at least half an hour.

2)   Apple and pear chutney with ginger and spices

Ingredients:
- **200 g of apples**
- **200 g of golden onions**
- **150 g of ripe but firm pears**
- **40 g of whole cane sugar**
- **the juice of ½ lemon**
- **140 ml of apple cider vinegar**
- **4 cm of freshly chopped ginger**
- **½ c of dried ginger powder**
- **½ c of powdered cumin**
- **100 ml of water, salt**

Peel and cut the apples and pears into small pieces. Gather them in a thick-bottomed saucepan with the peeled and thinly sliced onions; add the rest of the ingredients and mix. Cook over medium heat for about 40 minutes, stirring often. If necessary, wet with a little water. Continue cooking until you have reached the consistency of a jam. Pour the still warm chutney into the jars and consume it within a week, keeping it in the refrigerator anyway.

3)   Rice cream flavored with ginger, turmeric and cinnamon

Ingredients:
- **250 g of gluten free rice biscuits**
- **80 g toasted hazelnuts**
- **500 g rice milk**
- **40 g starch**
- **3 cm cinnamon**
- **8 g of fresh turmeric**
- **20 g fresh ginger**
- **70 g brown sugar**
- **500 g of clean pumpkin**
- **100 g of cane sugar**
- **3 cm cinnamon**
- **water q.s.**

Chop the biscuits and half of the hazelnuts. Heat the rice milk with the cinnamon, which you will then remove. Grate the turmeric and ginger, put them in a kitchen towel, and squeeze them in the milk. When the milk is hot, add the starch and sugar, stirring with a whisk, and cook until the cream has thickened. Let it cool down. Dice the pumpkin and put it in a saucepan with the sugar, cinnamon, and 33 cl of water. Cook until the pumpkin is soft, then blend it with the blender and let it cool. Compose the cake in layers, alternating the biscuits, compote, and cream. As a topping, use the remaining chopped hazelnuts.

4)   Beetroot brownies

Ingredients:
- **2 boiled beets**
- **200 g semi-wholemeal flour**
- **100 g dark chocolate (80-90%)**
- **50 g extra virgin olive oil**
- **50 g rice malt**
- **16 g yeast**
- **flaked almonds to taste**
- **1 handful of toasted hazelnuts**

Grate the beets, melt the chocolate in a bain-marie, add the oil, the malt, add the beets and mix everything. Add the sifted flour and baking powder. Mix well until the mixture is quite thick and soft. At this point, add the toasted hazelnuts and coarsely cut them with a knife. Transfer the dough to a previously greased square baking dish (about 30-40 cm). Bake in a preheated oven at 180 ° for about 30 minutes.

5)   Soft blueberry pie

Ingredients:
- **250 g semi-wholemeal flour**
- **200 g of soy drink**
- **Juice and grated zest of 1 lemon**
- **16 g yeast**
- **50 g extra virgin olive oil**
- **50 g rice malt**
- **1 pinch of salt**
- **250 g blueberries**

Gather the flour, yeast, salt, lemon zest in a bowl; mix everything. Combine the soy drink, lemon juice, oil, and malt. Stir well until you get a velvety, lump-free consistency. Now add the blueberries. Transfer the dough to a previously greased loaf pan (about 30 cm). Bake in a preheated oven at 180 ° for about 30-40 minutes. The toothpick test is recommended to verify internal cooking. Let the cake cool before enjoying it. Keep inside a container for three days.

6)   Lactose-free strawberry ice cream

Ingredients:
- **500 g of clean organic strawberries**
- **the juice of 1/2 lemon**
- **100 g of rice syrup**
- **260 ml of unsweetened rice milk**

Cut the strawberries, sprinkle them with the lemon juice and rice syrup, mix and let them rest in the refrigerator for half an hour.

After this time, blend the mixture briefly with the rice milk. Leave it to cool for another half hour. Operate the ice cream maker and pour the mixture. It will take between 20 and 25 minutes to get good ice cream, be divided into cups or glasses, and be enjoyed immediately.

7)   Coconut balls

Ingredients:
- **1 cup of cashews**
- **5 dates**
- **grated coconut to taste**
- **rice milk to taste**

Pitted the dates, cut them into small pieces, put them in a robot together with the cashews, and blended them finely. With your hands, form balls, compacting them well. Let them rest for half an hour in the fridge. Meanwhile, mix a little coconut with two tablespoons of rice milk. Take the balls back and roll them in this mixture until they are evenly covered. Finally, put them in the paper cups and serve them.

8)   Pear and cinnamon cake

Ingredients:
- **140 g of type 0 wheat flour**
- **160 g of millet flour**
- **1 p of sea salt**
- **½ teaspoon of yeast**
- **4 medium pears (2 quite ripe, 2 firmer)**
- **about 160 ml of rice milk**
- **100 ml of oil**
- **180 g of rice malt**
- **½ teaspoon of ground cinnamon**

Begin to heat the oven to 180 ° C. In the meantime, combine the wheat and millet flour in a bowl, the sea salt, yeast and mix well. Clean and peel the pears and cut only the two firmest into thin slices. Set the other two pears aside. Line a pan 20-22 cm in diameter with baking paper and arrange the pear slices on the bottom, overlapping them so that there are no gaps. Then cut the two more ripe pears into small pieces and place them in a mixer bowl. Add the rice milk, the oil, the malt, and the cinnamon and blend well until you obtain a smooth mixture which you will combine with the dry ingredients previously mixed, mixing briefly. Pour everything into the pan on the slices of pear. Bake and cook for 40-45 minutes. Finally, remove the cake from the oven, let it cool for 5-10 minutes before serving it with a vegetable cream sauce sweetened with a few tablespoons of rice malt of about.

9)   Vegan apple pie

Ingredients:
- **3 apples**
- **250 g of type 1 wheat flour**
- **60 g of raisins**
- **60 g of almonds**
- **About 250 ml of apple juice**
- **50 g of corn oil**
- **1 teaspoon of cinnamon**
- **grated lemon peel**
- **1/2 sachet of baking powder**
- **1 pinch of salt**

Soak the raisins. In a bowl, put the dry ingredients: flour, chopped almonds, lemon peel, cinnamon, and salt; stir with care. In another, gather the apple juice, the oil, the raisins, the peeled and chopped apples; mix them well, and mix them with the other container's contents. Mix the mixture carefully, roll it out in a pan; bake at 180 degrees for about 50-60 minutes. Check the cooking with a toothpick: if it comes out dry, turn off the oven. Let the cake rest briefly, unmold it, and let it cool completely on a wire rack before enjoying.

10) Carrot cake

Ingredients:
- **200 g of wholemeal flour**
- **80 g of almonds**
- **80 g of raisins**
- **200 g of carrots**
- **100 g of rice malt**
- **4 tablespoons of sunflower oil**
- **1 orange**
- **3 tablespoons of corn starch**
- **1 teaspoon of yeast**
- **½ teaspoon of natural vanilla**
- **soya milk**
- **1 pinch of salt**

Wash the orange, grate the zest and squeeze the juice. Put the first in a bowl together with the flour, finely ground almonds, starch, yeast, vanilla, and salt. Stir. Mix the oil, malt, and orange juice in a bowl. Gradually add them to the dry ingredients. Complete with grated carrots and rinsed raisins. If the dough is too firm, dilute it with a little soy milk. Line a square mold of about 20 cm on each side with baking paper. Transfer the mixture, level it, and bake at 180 degrees for about 45 minutes. Check the cooking with a toothpick, which must come out dry. Let the cake cool in the pan, turn it out of the mold, and let it cool.

11) Baked stuffed apples

Ingredients:
- **6 apples**
- **1 orange**
- **¾ cup of shelled walnuts**
- **¾ cup of raisins**
- **¼ cup of natural apple juice**
- **1 tablespoon of miso**

Wash and with a knife, starting from the top of the apple, make room for the filling. Heat the oven to 150 °. Rinse the raisins and chop them with the walnuts. Wash the orange and finely grate the zest. Add the orange zest, miso, and a teaspoon to the raisin and nut mixture. Mix well. Stuff the apples with the dough. Arrange the apples in a baking dish. Pierce them with a fork all around so that they do not explode during cooking. Pour the apple and orange juice into the pan and bake in the oven for half an hour. Eat them warm or cold.

12) Orange cake

Ingredients:
- **300 g of wheat flour 00**
- **150 g of clear raw cane sugar**
- **½ sachet of yeast**
- **the zest and juice of an orange**
- **50 ml of extra virgin olive oil**
- **vanilla sugar to taste**

In a bowl, mix flour, brown sugar, yeast, the grated rind of an orange together with its juice, extra virgin olive oil, and about 100 ml of water. Mix everything with an electric or hand whisk until you get a creamy mixture. Transfer to a pan greased with oil and sprinkled with flour. Bake at 180 degrees for half an hour. When cooked, spread the icing sugar over the cake.

Chapter 11: Sauces, toppings and condiments

1)   Black Cabbage Pesto

Ingredients:
- **350 g of black cabbage**
- **50 g of walnut kernels**
- **1 heaping tablespoon of pine nuts**
- **1 clove of garlic**
- **5 tablespoons of oil**
- **a pinch of salt**

Clean and steam the cabbage for 5-6 minutes. Blend it with the walnuts, garlic, pine nuts, oil, and salt, helping you if needed with a little water kept aside. It was excellent for dressing pasta, cereals, rice, and polenta, filling for crepes, sandwiches, and savory scones, or simply spreading on croutons for an unusual and tasty appetizer.

2)   Curry tofu cream

Ingredients:
- **300 g of tofu**
- **1 onion**
- **1 apple**
- **1 teaspoon of spicy curry**
- **2 teaspoons of sweet curry**
- **vegetable broth**
- **3 tablespoons of oil**
- **salt**

Finely chop the onion and put it in a pan covered with broth. Cook it over low heat, with the lid on, until it is soft. If necessary, gradually add more hot broth. Meanwhile, put the tofu in a saucepan, cover it with water and let it boil slowly. Turn off the heat and let it cool. Wash the apple and core it, cut it into wedges and add it to the onion. Mix the two types of curry in a little broth and pour them into the pan. Stir well and cook for another 5 minutes. Turn off the heat and let it rest. Combine the diced tofu and the curry sauce in a blender. Add the oil and a little salt. Blend them until smooth, helping you if needed with a little broth. When the sauce is creamy, serve it spread on bread, or use it to season cooked cereals or vegetables.

3)   Yogurt mayonnaise

Ingredients:
- **200 g of soy yogurt**
- **oil, lemon juice**
- **1 pinch of mustard powder**
- **salt**

Put the yogurt in a container with high sides. It will gradually pour in the oil (one tablespoon at a time, it will take four to five) and whip the sauce with the hand blender. When the mayonnaise is thick, add a few drops of lemon juice, mustard, and salt. Leave it in the fridge for a couple of hours before enjoying it with a vegetable salad or roasted vegetables.

4)   Aubergine sauce

Ingredients:
- **2 medium-sized aubergine**
- **1 clove of garlic**
- **abundant basil**
- **1 sprig of parsley**
- **a pinch of grated lemon zest**
- **20 g of pine nuts**
- **extra virgin olive oil**
- **whole sea salt**

In a saucepan, bring lightly salted water to a boil. In the meantime, clean, peel and divide the aubergine pulp into chunks. Blanch the aubergines for 3 minutes, then blend them until they are reduced to a smooth and homogeneous cream. Season with salt and season with oil and a small piece of lemon zest. With a mixer's help, prepare an emulsified sauce based on garlic, basil, a few parsley leaves, extra virgin olive oil, and salt. Serve the aubergine sauce with the basil emulsion and the pine nuts toasted in a pan on top.

5)   Ginger and avocado sauce

Ingredients:
- 2 ripe avocados
- the juice of 1 lemon
- 1 clove of garlic
- 2 tablespoons of chopped walnuts
- 1 tablespoon of fresh grated ginger
- 1 pinch of salt
- 125 grams of soy yogurt

Peel the avocados and pit them. Mash the pulp with a fork and sprinkle it immediately with the filtered lemon juice to prevent it from blackening. Add the crushed garlic and grated ginger. Finally, gently stir in the yogurt and add salt. To speed up the timing, you can put everything in the mixer.

6) Zucchini pesto

Ingredients:
- **Zucchini 200 g**
- **Extra virgin olive oil 125 g**
- **Salt up to 2 g**
- **Pine nuts 30 g**
- **Parmesan to grate 60 g**
- **Basil 10 g**

Wash the zucchini, remove the ends, and chop them with the help of a grater with large holes. Place the grated zucchini in a colander, salt them lightly and let them rest for 30 minutes so that they lose the excess liquid. Then pour them into the mixer with the pine nuts and basil leaves previously cleaned with a dry cloth. Add the grated Parmesan and a part of the oil. Then turn on the mixer and blend for a few seconds. Add the rest of the oil and blend until you get a smooth cream. Transfer the mixture to a bowl and use the zucchini pesto according to your needs.

7)   Rocket pesto

Ingredients:
- **Rocket 100 g**
- **Extra virgin olive oil 150 g**
- **Pine nuts 50 g**
- **Parmesan to grate 100 g**
- **1 clove garlic**
- **Salt up to taste**

Wash the rocket very well, dry it, and put it in the cup of a mixer: also add the pine nuts, the parmesan; add the whole peeled clove of garlic and salt. At this point, add a small part of the olive oil. Begin to blend everything at low speed and add the remaining olive oil gradually until you get a well combined and fluid cream.

8) Yogurt Based Sauce

Ingredients:

- **250 g of Greek yogurt**
- **1 teaspoon of freeze-dried garlic**
- **1 teaspoon of lemon juice**
- **1 tablespoon of extra virgin olive oil**
- **basil**
- **mint**
- **dill**
- **salt**
- **pepper**

Pour the Greek yogurt into a bowl and add the freeze-dried garlic, lemon juice, salt, and pepper. Mix everything, then add the chopped herbs and oil. Stir and keep in the fridge to flavor at least half an hour before serving the yogurt sauce to accompany your dishes.

9)   Fresh tomato sauce with basil

Ingredients:
- **Copper tomatoes 1.2 kg**
- **Extra virgin olive oil 3 tbsp**
- **Salt up to taste**
- **Basil 8 leaves**

Remove the stalks and wash them very well, then dry them. Cut each tomato into two halves and remove the green part of each of them' stem. Squeeze the two halves of the tomato into a bowl or sink so that all the seeds come out. Put the tomatoes in a steel pot, which you will arrange on low heat covered by the lid; let the tomatoes cook, turning them from time to time until they are wilted and come apart. Pass the tomatoes with a vegetable mill making the sauce converge in a bowl; once all the tomatoes have been passed, pour the sauce into a smaller steel pot that you will put on the stove. Add the salt and oil to the sauce, consume it over high heat to the desired density, turn off the heat, and add the whole basil or coarsely chopped by hand. Perfect with spaghetti!

10) Guacamole

Ingredients:

- **Ripe avocado 1**
- **Green chilli 1**
- **Copper tomatoes 1**
- **Extra virgin olive oil 20 g**
- **Lime juice 10 g**
- **Shallot 10 g**
- **Black pepper 1 pinch**
- **Salt up to 1 pinch**

Start by looking after the avocado. Cut it in half lengthwise, then sink the knife's blade into the core and pull to extract it easily. Cut the pulp with a small knife to remove it more easily with a spoon; collect it in a small bowl. Then cut the lime in half and squeeze it to obtain the juice, be poured on the avocado pulp; Then, season with salt and pepper, and mash the pulp with a fork. Set aside, then peel and finely chop the shallot, then wash, dry, and slice the tomato: obtained from the cubes' slices. Then tick the green (or red) chili pepper, empty it of its seeds, cut it into strips, and then into cubes. Then in the bowl with the crushed avocado pulp, pour the chopped shallot and the diced tomatoes. Also, add the chili and oil, stir and add more salt and pepper if necessary. Your guacamole sauce is ready to be enjoyed!

11) Green sauce

Ingredients:

- **Anchovies in oil fillets 3**
- **2 cloves garlic**
- **Parsley 120 g**
- **Salted capers 1 tbsp**
- **Firm yolks 2**
- **White wine vinegar 50 g**
- **Stale bread (only the crumb) 80 g**
- **Extra virgin olive oil 150 g**
- **Black pepper to taste**
- **Salt up to taste**

Heat the water in a pan and as soon as the water is boiling, dip the eggs to be covered with water and cook them for about 8-9 minutes, then let them cool for a few moments before peeling them. Finally, sift the egg yolks into a bowl. Then remove the crust from the bread and cut the crumb into pieces that you will pour into a bowl together with the wine vinegar. Leave to soak for about ten minutes. Meanwhile, peel, divide in half and remove the garlic's core, to say the central part. Desalt the capers by repeatedly rinsing them under running water and chop them together with the garlic and anchovies, passing the blade over the mince to crush it well to obtain a well-blended paste that you will pour into the bowl with the yolk. Squeeze the crumb with your hands and add it to the bowl. Finally, finely chop the parsley leaves, well washed and dried, and pour these into the bowl along with a pinch of salt and pepper. Mix thoroughly and sprinkle with extra virgin olive oil. Let it rest at room temperature for a couple of hours, and your green sauce is ready to accompany your favorite dishes, from boiled meats to fish to croutons!

12) Broccoli pesto

Ingredients:
- **Broccoli 320 g**
- **Pine nuts (shelled) 30 g**
- **Peeled almonds 10 g**
- **Parmesan to grate 30 g**
- **Basil 10 g**
- **Extra virgin olive oil 70 g**
- **Salt up to 1 pinch**

Wash the broccoli, divide the florets from the central stem and let them blanch for 5 minutes, then drain and pour them into a bowl filled with water and ice to let them cool and keep the color alive. When the broccoli has cooled, drain it from the ice water and dry it with a paper towel. Transfer the broccoli to the mixer, add the basil leaves, the peeled almonds, the pine nuts, the grated Parmesan cheese, and half of the extra virgin olive oil. Operate the blades to blend all the ingredients and add the remaining oil; if the mixture is too dry, add more oil. The pesto must be creamy; once ready, you can use it to season pasta.

Conclusion

About 20-40% of American adults "suffer" from fatty liver disease. Due to its asymptomaticity, more than 90% of people with fatty liver occasionally discover this disorder. This is why hepatic steatosis is often discovered by accident, during an ultrasound performed for simple control or another pathology. However, slight increases in transaminases (enzymes present in the blood) are often indicators of fatty liver disease. At the same time, fatigue, weakness, sudden weight loss can be signs of more advanced disease. In itself, this disorder is not an actual disease but a simple metabolic disadvantage. Fatty liver disease or fatty liver disease is a condition characterized, as the name suggests, by the presence of fat within the liver. The causes of this can be different, such as some diseases such as diabetes, metabolic syndrome, anemia, and an incorrect diet, which can lead to the onset of this condition over time. The fatty liver diet involves the exclusion of a large variety of foods that could worsen liver health. The therapeutic approach for fatty liver disease consists of lifestyle modification and proper nutrition.

www.ingramcontent.com/pod-product-compliance
Lightning Source LLC
Chambersburg PA
CBHW061315120726
48001CB00002B/514